THE AUTHORS

Robert H. Whitaker MD, MChir, FRCS graduated from the University of Cambridge and trained at University College Hospital, London. He spent a year at Johns Hopkins Hospital, Baltimore, in the Urological Research Laboratories before returning to continue his training first at the St Peters Hospital group in London then as a Senior Lecturer in Urology at the London Hospital Medical School. He was appointed as a Consultant Urologist at Addenbrooke's Hospital in Cambridge in 1973 and spent 20 years practising mostly paediatric urology before retiring from clinical practice to join the Department of Anatomy in Cambridge to help with the teaching of students and trainee surgeons.

Neil R. Borley MB, BS, FRCS trained at Guy's Hospital, London and after performing house jobs in medicine and surgery there he embarked upon a career in surgery. He undertook a surgical rotation at Addenbrooke's Hospital, Cambridge, before becoming a Demonstrator in the Department of Anatomy in Cambridge under Professor Harold Ellis. He passed the Primary FRCS examination in 1993 for which he received the Hallet Prize and then continued his surgical training at Papworth Hospital and Kent and Canterbury Hospital. After moving to Oxford as Surgical Registrar, he is now Clinical Lecturer in Surgery and Clinical Tutor in the Nuffield Department of Surgery, Oxford.

We would welcome and value any reader feedback. Let us know how you think this approach could be improved by emailing us at the following email address: authors@blacksci.co.uk.

INSTANT ANATOMY

INSTANT ANATOMY

Robert H. Whitaker
MD, MChir, FRCS
Department of Anatomy
University of Cambridge

Neil R. Borley
MB, BS, FRCS, FRCS (ed)
Nuffield Department of Surgery
University of Oxford

SECOND EDITION

Blackwell
Science

© 2000 by Blackwell Science Ltd
a Blackwell Publishing company

Editorial Offices:
Blackwell Science Ltd, 9600 Garsington Road, Oxford OX4 2DQ, UK
    Tel: +44 (0)1865 776868
Blackwell Publishing Inc., 350 Main Street, Malden, MA 02148-5020, USA
    Tel: +1 781 388 8250
Blackwell Science Asia Pty, 550 Swanston Street, Carlton, Victoria 3053, Australia
    Tel: +61 (0)3 8359 1011

First published 1994
Second edition 2000
Reprinted 2001, 2004

Library of Congress Cataloging-in-Publication Data

Whitaker, R. H. (Robert H.)
    Instant anatomy/Robert H. Whitaker,
    Neil R. Borley. — 2nd ed.
        p.   cm.
    ISBN 0-632-05403-4
    1. Human anatomy
    Outlines, syllabi, etc.
    I. Borley, Neil R.
    II. Title.
    QM31.W55   2000
    611—dc21

                                                     99–39812
                                                        CIP

ISBN 0-632-05403-4

A catalogue record for this title is available from the British Library

Set by Graphicraft Limited, Hong Kong
Printed and bound in India using acid-free paper
by Replika Press Pvt. Ltd., Kundli 131 028

For further information on Blackwell Publishing, visit our website:
www.blackwellpublishing.com

CONTENTS

PREFACE TO SECOND EDITION

We have been pleasantly surprised at the success of this book and most grateful to all the students and colleagues who have made constructive criticisms. There were a number of errors of fact, expression and omission in the original text and we very much hope that most of these have been corrected.

We have resisted the temptation of those who suggested that we illustrate each muscle as such information can be found in other larger texts and we fear for the loss of the compactness that seems so popular with students. We have, however, expanded the section on the autonomic system, particularly in respect to the head and neck and abdomen as these remain areas of wonderment in the minds of many students, and we suspect others as well (!) but they are, of course, important clinically in respect to basic neurological and abdominal examinations. We have included our favourite lateral view of the cavernous sinus as we believe that it adds considerably to the conventional coronal view that appears in all the textbooks and improved our understanding of this important area. We may be criticised for giving excessive space for what might appear to some as less important aspects of anatomy but we have done this because we are so aware of the difficulty that some students have with learning these topics or even finding the information concisely in larger texts.

We remain committed to teaching anatomy to a high standard even if limited in the degree of complexity that has now been imposed on us by modern views on core courses for students and dictated by those who make the rules for surgical trainees.

We hope that this second edition will prove useful and be an inspiration for some young surgeons.

ROBERT WHITAKER
NEIL BORLEY
Cambridge and Oxford, 2000

PREFACE TO FIRST EDITION

How many times have you looked up the course of an artery or nerve in one of the excellent anatomy textbooks that are available today only to find that the details are spread over several sections of the book and that an instant summary is not available? At times like this you wish there was a quick reference book with all the answers neatly catalogued in dictionary format.

We have attempted to provide such a concise text for rapid reference. Of course, we emphasise that this is not a text for learning anatomy from scratch but one that should be used in conjunction with one of the fuller texts that has stood the test of time. The book is designed for those who already have some working knowledge of anatomy and need to find accurate facts quickly.

Both authors have been sufficiently recent students of anatomy for higher degrees and for teaching undergraduate medical students that each can remember the problems that both students and they themselves encountered. The book has been compiled with this in mind.

It is designed primarily for undergraduate medical students and prospective surgeons who are studying for a higher degree in surgery. For each of these groups we believe it will be ideal. However, it should also be extremely useful for all clinicians who need to remind themselves of anatomical facts at all stages in their careers and for other professional groups such as nurses, physiotherapists and radiographers.

Inevitably in a book of this size there has been some selection of material for inclusion and no attempt has been made to provide details of minutiae that appear in the fuller texts.

The authors' original artwork was redrawn with a graphics program by Jane Fallows, medical illustrator, to whom the authors owe an immense debt of gratitude for her skill and patience.

ROBERT WHITAKER
NEIL BORLEY
Cambridge, 1994

NOTES ON THE TEXT

The illustrations show the **right** side of the body as viewed from in front, unless otherwise indicated. The two exceptions are the cervical and brachial plexuses where it makes little difference as to which side they are viewed and they are more conveniently drawn and remembered as they are shown here. Where there might be confusion, a small compass has been added to indicate the left and right *sides of the body*.

Eponymous names appear sparingly and only when they are in common usage. The following abbreviations have been used as appropriate throughout the text.

List of abbreviations

ant	anterior(ly)
art(s)	artery(ies)
br(s)	branch(s)
CMC	carpometacarpal
div(s)	division(s)
ext	external
inf	inferior(ly)
int	internal
IP	interphalangeal
jnt(s)	joint(s)
lat	lateral(ly)
lig(s)	ligament(s)
med	medial(ly)
MC(s)	metacarpal(s)
MCP	metacarpophalangeal
MTP	metatarsophalangeal
MT(s)	metatarsal(s)
N(s) or n(s)	nerve(s)
post	posterior(ly)
prox	proximal
sup	superior(ly)
TMT	tarsometatarsal
V(s)	vein(s)

Note: Abbreviations are not used for muscle names or in titles. The following words are always written in full: greater, lesser, middle, superficial and combinations such as mediolateral.

1: ARTERIES

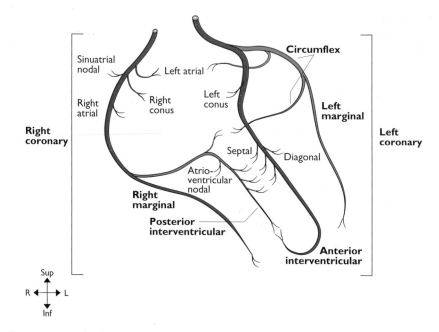

Coronary arteries

I

CORONARY ARTERIES
From: Ascending aorta
To: Myocardium

Right coronary artery. Originates from the anterior (new nomenclature: right) aortic sinus. It passes anteriorly between the pulmonary trunk and the right auricle to reach the atrioventricular sulcus in which it runs down the anterior surface of the right cardiac border and then onto the inferior surface of the heart. It terminates at the junction of the atrioventricular sulcus and the posterior interventricular groove by anastomosing with the circumflex branch of the left coronary artery and giving off the posterior interventricular (posterior descending) artery. It supplies the right atrium and part of the left atrium, the sinuatrial node in 60% of cases, the right ventricle, the posterior part of the inter-ventricular septum and the atrioventricular node in 80% of cases.

Left coronary artery. Arises from the left posterior (new nomenclature: left) aortic sinus. It passes laterally, posterior to the pulmonary trunk and anterior to the left auricle to reach the atrioventricular groove where it divides into an anterior interventricular (formally left anterior descending) artery and circumflex branches. The circumflex artery runs in the atrio-ventricular sulcus around the left border of the heart to anastomose with the right coronary artery. The anterior inter-ventricular artery descends on the anterior surface of the heart in the anterior interventricular groove and around the apex of the heart into the posterior interven-tricular groove where it anastomoses with the posterior interventricular branch of the right coronary artery. The left coronary artery supplies the left atrium, left ventricle, anterior interventricular septum, sinuatrial node in 40% of cases and the atrioven-tricular node in 20%.

Dominance. In approximately 10% of hearts the posterior interventricular artery arises from the circumflex artery (left coronary) and then most of the left ventricle and interventricular septum are supplied by the left coronary artery. The heart is said to have *left cardiac dominance.*

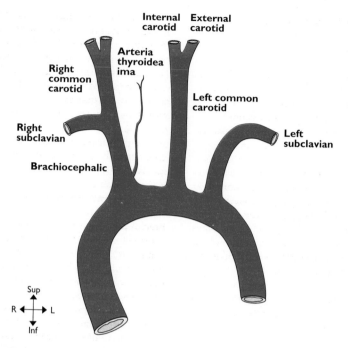

Ascending & arch of aorta

ASCENDING & ARCH OF AORTA
From: Left ventricle
To: Descending aorta

Ascending aorta. Arises at the vestibule of the left ventricle at the level of the third left costal cartilage and passes upwards and slightly to the right to a point behind the sternum at the level of the manubriosternal joint (second costal cartilage) where it becomes the arch of the aorta. It is enclosed in fibrous and serous pericardium. Anterior to it are the right auricle, the infundibulum of the right ventricle and pulmonary trunk. Posterior, lie the left atrium, the right pulmonary artery and right main bronchus. To the left lie the pulmonary trunk and the left auricle. To the right are the superior vena cava and the right atrium.

Arch of aorta. The arch begins posterior to the manubriosternal joint at the level of the second costal cartilage and passes posterior and to the left, over the left main bronchus to end at the left side of the body of T4 vertebra. Its highest level is the mid point of the manubrium sterni and at this level its three main branches emerge. Anterior and to the left of the arch are (from anterior to posterior) the left phrenic nerve, vagal and sympathetic contributions to the cardiac plexus, and the left vagus. Also, the left superior intercostal vein runs forwards on the arch anterior to the vagus and posterior to the phrenic nerve. Lateral to all these structures are the pleura and left lung. Posterior and to the right of the arch are the trachea, deep cardiac plexus, left recurrent laryngeal nerve, oesophagus, thoracic duct and the body of T4. Inferior to the arch are the pulmonary bifurcation, the left main bronchus, the ligamentum arteriosum and the left recurrent laryngeal nerve. From its superior surface emerge the brachiocephalic artery, the left common carotid and left subclavian arteries. Within the adventitia of the ascending and arch of the aorta lie baro- and chemoreceptors.

Brachiocephalic artery. Arises from the convexity of the aortic arch behind the manubrium sterni and passes upwards and posteriorly to the right. It divides into the right subclavian and right common carotid arteries posterior to the right sternoclavicular joint. Anterior to it are the left brachiocephalic vein with the right inferior thyroid vein entering it, and the thymic remnants. The artery initially lies anterior to the trachea then passes to lie on its right lateral side. On the right of the artery are the right brachiocephalic vein, upper part of the superior vena cava, the pleura and the cardiac branches of the vagus. The main vagal trunk is more posterolateral. At the origin of the brachiocephalic artery the left common carotid artery lies posteriorly on its left.

continued

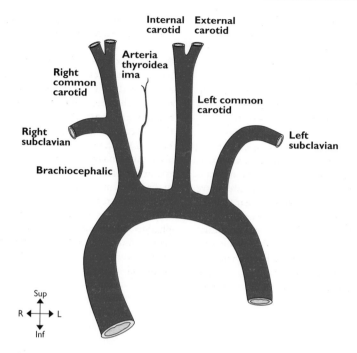

Ascending & arch of aorta

Common carotid arteries. The right common carotid artery arises from the brachiocephalic artery as it divides posterior to the right sternoclavicular joint, whilst the left common carotid arises from the convexity of the aortic arch. Both end as the arteries bifurcate at the level of the upper border of the thyroid cartilage (C4).

Left common carotid artery (thorax). Lying anterior to the thoracic part of this artery are the left brachiocephalic vein and the thymic remnant. Posterior to it in its lower part are the left subclavian artery and the trachea whilst further superiorly there is the left recurrent laryngeal nerve, the thoracic duct and the left side of the oesophagus. On its right at its origin is the brachiocephalic artery but as it ascends the inferior thyroid veins and the trachea come to lie on its right side. To its left lie the vagus, the left phrenic nerve and the left pleura and lung.

Both common carotid arteries (cervical). Ascend in the neck slightly laterally from a point posterior to the sternoclavicular joint to end at the level of the upper border of the thyroid cartilage (C4) at which point there is a dilatation—the carotid sinus (a baroreceptor). On the posterior aspect of the bifurcation there is the carotid body (a chemoreceptor). Lying between left and right arteries, and medial to each, progressively from below are the trachea, recurrent laryngeal nerves, thyroid gland, larynx and pharynx. Each artery lies in its carotid sheath with the internal jugular vein lateral to it and the vagus nerve between and posterior to them both.

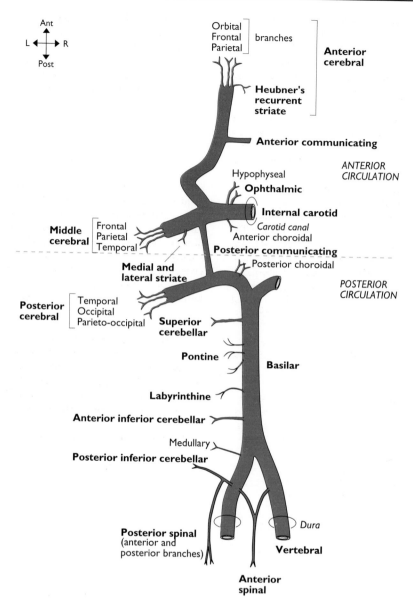

Internal carotid, vertebrobasilar system & circle of Willis
Note: (1) Labyrinthine usually arises from anterior inferior cerebellar; (2) posterior spinal may come from vertebral

INTERNAL CAROTID ARTERY, VERTEBROBASILAR SYSTEM & CIRCLE OF WILLIS
From: Bifurcation of the common carotid
   arts (C4) & first parts of subclavian arts
To: Terminal brs

The internal carotid artery angles from the bifurcation slightly posteriorly to reach the carotid canal through which it enters the skull to end as middle and anterior cerebral arteries. At its origin it possesses a dilatation in which lie the carotid sinus and body. In the neck it is crossed laterally by, from below up, the pharyngeal branch of the vagus (X), glossopharyngeal nerve (IX), stylopharyngeus and styloglossus. It lies on the pharyngeal wall and the pharyngobasilar fascia. Within the carotid canal it turns 90 degrees anteromedially to run through the petrous temporal bone where it lies medial to the middle ear. It then turns 90 degrees superiorly to pass across the upper limit of the foramen lacerum. It then turns 90 degrees anteriorly to pass forwards, lateral to the body of the sphenoid which it grooves. Here it lies in the medial wall of the cavernous sinus with the abducent nerve (VI) on its lateral side. At the anterior end of the cavernous sinus it turns 90 degrees superiorly then 90 degrees posteriorly to pass medial to the anterior clinoid process and lateral to the pituitary stalk and optic chiasma. It ends as terminal branches on the medial surface of the temporal lobe.

Anterior cerebral artery is formed by the bifurcation of the internal carotid artery. It passes anteriorly over the optic nerve to arch over the genu of the corpus callosum on the medial aspect of the cerebral hemispheres where it ends as terminal branches.

Middle cerebral artery is formed by the bifurcation of the internal carotid artery. It runs laterally into the sylvian fissure then posterosuperiorly in the sulcus where it divides into terminal branches.

Basilar artery is formed by the junction of the left and right vertebral arteries (see subclavian artery, pp. 16–19) anterior to the upper medulla. From there it ascends lying angled forwards between the pons and the clivus in a slight depression on the anterior surface of the pons. It terminates at the upper border of the pons as posterior cerebral arteries.

Posterior cerebral artery is formed by the bifurcation of the basilar artery. It passes laterally around the cerebral peduncle to run posteriorly above the tentorium cerebelli on the inferomedial surface of the occipital lobe where it divides into terminal branches.

(Other branches of the internal carotid artery, not illustrated, are caroticotympanic, pterygoid and cavernous arteries.)

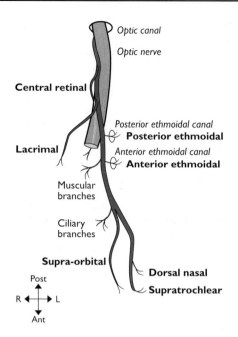

Ophthalmic artery
Note: Right side viewed from above

OPHTHALMIC ARTERY
From: Internal carotid art
To: Terminal brs in orbit

It arises from the internal carotid artery as it lies medial to the anterior clinoid process and runs anteriorly through the optic canal within the optic nerve's dural sheath, lying inferolateral to the nerve. Small branches supply the proximal nerve. In the orbit the artery leaves the dural sheath and passes forwards around the lateral side of the nerve to cross anterior to it to reach the medial orbit. It then continues medially between superior oblique and medial rectus to pass out of the cone of muscles to reach the medial wall of the orbit. The artery continues forwards to terminate at the medial orbital border deep to the superior tarsal plate as branches which leave the orbit to anastomose with branches of the facial artery.

Central retinal artery. This small, important end artery supplies the optic nerve and retina. It leaves the ophthalmic artery below the optic nerve and then, half way along the orbital part of the optic nerve, enters first the dural sheath and then the nerve itself.

(Other branches, not illustrated, (1) of ophthalmic artery are anterior meningeal and medial palpebral arteries; (2) of lacrimal artery are lateral palpebral, zygomatic and recurrent meningeal arteries; (3) of muscular is anterior ciliary artery.)

Ant - clinoid process

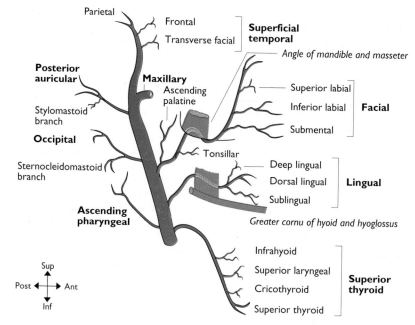

External carotid artery

EXTERNAL CAROTID ARTERY
From: Upper border of thyroid cartilage (C4)
To: Terminal brs within parotid gland post
   to neck of mandible

The artery arises within the carotid sheath from the bifurcation of the common carotid artery. It lies at first anteromedial to the internal carotid artery but spirals over it to come to lie lateral to it at the level of C2. Initially, it angles slightly forwards then curves backwards as it ascends to enter the parotid gland between deep and superficial lobes. During its course it is crossed by, from below upwards: the upper root of the ansa cervicalis, the hypoglossal nerve, the posterior belly of digastric, stylohyoid, the stylohyoid ligament and the facial nerve (within the parotid). Passing between it and the internal carotid artery are, from below upwards, the pharyngeal branch of the vagus (X), glossopharyngeal nerve (IX), stylopharyngeus and styloglossus. It lies on, from below upwards, pharyngeal wall, superior laryngeal branch of the vagus (X) and deep parotid lobe.

Superior thyroid artery.
Arises from the anterior surface of the external carotid artery near its origin and runs inferiorly and forwards deep to omohyoid and lateral to the inferior constrictor and external laryngeal nerve to reach the upper pole of the thyroid gland.

Lingual artery.
Runs superiorly looping over the greater cornu of the hyoid bone and passes medially (deep) to hyoglossus then into the substance of the tongue.

Facial artery.
Arises from the anteromedial surface of the external carotid artery and runs above the hyoid bone deep to digastric and passes upwards to reach the posterior surface of the submandibular gland which it grooves deeply, lying medial to the body of the mandible. Here it lies on superior constrictor, directly lateral to the palatine tonsil. It then follows a tortuous course looping at first inferiorly then upwards around the lower border of the mandible to cross the bone anterior to the insertion of masseter (where it is easily palpable). It then runs in the superficial tissues of the face towards the angle of the mouth where it turns superiorly towards the medial canthus of the eye. (Other branches, not illustrated, are glandular (to submandibular gland) and lateral nasal arteries.)

Superficial temporal artery.
Runs superiorly between the deep and superficial lobes of the parotid gland, over the posterior end of the zygomatic process (where it is easily palpable) and terminates in the subcutaneous tissues of the lateral scalp.

Maxillary artery

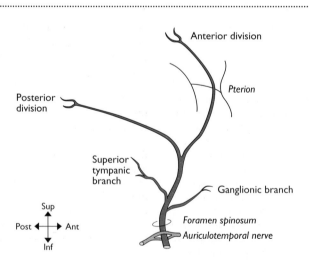

Middle meningeal artery

MAXILLARY ARTERY
From: **External carotid within parotid gland**
To: **Terminal brs in pterygopalatine fossa**

It arises from the external carotid artery within the parotid gland posterior to the neck of the mandible and ends as the sphenopalatine artery. The artery is divided into three portions by its relationship posterior, in, or anterior to the lateral pterygoid muscle. The first part passes deep to the neck of the mandible between the bone and the sphenomandibular ligament and runs anteriorly lateral to the inferior alveolar nerve to reach the border of the lateral pterygoid. The second part angles anteromedially between the two heads of lateral pterygoid between anterior and posterior divisions of the mandibular nerve. The third part leaves the lateral pterygoid to enter the pterygopalatine fossa where it terminates as branches which accompany the branches of the maxillary division of the trigeminal nerve (Vb).

Inferior alveolar artery. Passes inferolaterally posterior to the inferior alveolar nerve onto the medial surface of the ramus of the mandible which it grooves as it enters the inferior alveolar (mandibular) foramen in the mandible. It is distributed along the mandibular canal to the lower jaw and teeth. Its terminal branch appears as the mental branch through the mental foramen.

(Other branches, not illustrated, (1) of maxillary artery (third part) is artery of pterygoid canal; (2) of inferior alveolar artery are dental and mental; (3) of infraorbital artery are dental and anterior superior alveolar; (4) of posterior superior alveolar artery is dental.)

MIDDLE MENINGEAL ARTERY
From: **First part of maxillary art**
To: **Terminal brs**

It arises from the superomedial surface of the maxillary (first part) to run between the two rootlets of the auriculotemporal nerve as it passes vertically into the foramen spinosum in the greater wing of the sphenoid bone. After a very short course laterally over the greater wing of the sphenoid in the middle cranial fossa it divides into anterior and posterior divisions. The anterior division runs anterolaterally on the floor of the middle cranial fossa beneath the dura mater and grooves the greater wing of the sphenoid as it passes upwards to the junction of the lesser and greater wings. Here it may groove deeply or tunnel through the bone at the apex of the greater wing. It passes across the inner aspect of the pterion onto the parietal bone. The posterior division runs almost horizontally posterolateral over the inner aspect of the squamous temporal bone onto the lower parietal bone where it gives terminal branches.

Because of the problem of extradural haemorrhage caused by damage to this artery, the surface anatomy is important. Anterior branch: 3 cm above mid point of zygomatic arch. Posterior branch: on a line vertically from the mastoid process and horizontal from the upper margin of the orbit.

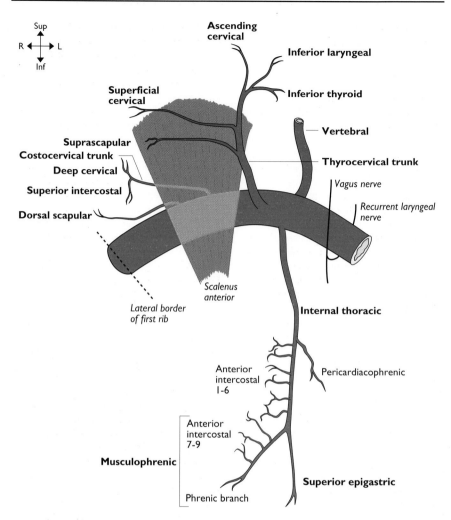

Sup
R ←+→ L
Inf

Ascending cervical

Inferior laryngeal

Superficial cervical

Inferior thyroid

Suprascapular
Costocervical trunk
Deep cervical
Superior intercostal

Dorsal scapular

Vertebral

Thyrocervical trunk

Vagus nerve

Recurrent laryngeal nerve

Scalenus anterior

Lateral border of first rib

Internal thoracic

Anterior intercostal 1-6

Pericardiacophrenic

Anterior intercostal 7-9

Musculophrenic

Superior epigastric

Phrenic branch

Subclavian artery

Note: (1) The superficial cervical artery is named 'transverse cervical artery' if it gives origin to the dorsal scapular artery instead of the latter arising separately from the second part of the subclavian artery; (2) phrenic branch of musculophrenic artery anastomoses with inferior phrenic artery

SUBCLAVIAN ARTERY

From: Right—brachiocephalic trunk
     Left—aortic arch
To: Axillary art

The subclavian arteries arise as indicated above and end at the outer border of the first rib where they become the axillary arteries. They each have three parts: (1) medial (three branches); (2) behind (two branches); and (3) lateral (no branches) to scalenus anterior.

Right subclavian artery—first part. Arises from the brachiocephalic artery behind the right sternoclavicular joint, lying initially posterior to the right common carotid artery, then passing upwards and laterally to reach the medial side of scalenus anterior. Anterior to this first part are the vagus (X), its cardiac branches, sympathetic nerves, the internal jugular and vertebral veins. The ansa subclavia (sympathetic nerves) curls around the artery to lie both anterior and posterior to it. As the artery arches laterally the suprapleural membrane and the right recurrent laryngeal nerve lie inferior and posterior to it.

Left subclavian artery—first part. Arises from the arch of the aorta just posterior and slightly to the left of the origin of the left common carotid artery at the level of the intervertebral disc of T3/T4. It passes upwards and then, behind the left sterno-clavicular joint, it arches laterally over the suprapleural membrane to the medial edge of scalenus anterior. Anterior to it in the thorax are the left common carotid artery, the left brachiocephalic vein, the left vagus and its cardiac branches and the left phrenic nerve. Posterior to it lie the left side of the oesophagus, the thoracic duct and longus colli. Medial to it is the trachea, the left recurrent laryngeal nerve and, more superiorly, the thoracic duct. In the neck it is crossed anteriorly by the left phrenic nerve and the thoracic duct.

Subclavian artery—second part. Lies posterior to scalenus anterior and anterior to scalenus medius. Anterior to scalenus anterior are the phrenic nerve and, slightly inferior, the subclavian vein. Postero-inferior are the suprapleural membrane and the lower trunk of the brachial plexus. Superior to it are the upper and middle trunks of the brachial plexus.

Subclavian artery—third part. Begins at the lateral margin of scalenus anterior and extends to the outer (lateral) margin of the first rib where it becomes the axillary artery. Anterior to it is the external jugular vein and its tributaries. Antero-inferior is the subclavian vein. Postero-inferior is the lower trunk of the brachial plexus and the first rib. Posterosuperior are the upper and middle trunks of the brachial plexus.

Vertebral artery (see also internal carotid, vertebrobasilar system & circle of Willis, pp. 8–9). Arises from the posterosuperior aspect of the first part of the subclavian artery and ends where the arteries from the two sides join to form the basilar artery at the lower pons. It angles posteriorly between the medial border of scalenus anterior and the lateral border of longus colli in the apex of the pyramidal space before entering the foramen in the transverse process of C6 behind its anterior tubercle (carotid tubercle of Chassaignac). Lying anterior to this first part are the common carotid artery and the vertebral vein and, more medially, the inferior thyroid artery and middle cervical ganglion. On the left the thoracic duct crosses it anteriorly. Posterior to it are the anterior primary rami of C7 and C8 nerves and more medially the inferior cervical (stellate) ganglion. The second part of the artery ascends within the foramina of the transverse processes of C6 to C1, accompanied by sympathetic nerves and vertebral veins. It passes out posteriorly behind the lateral mass of the atlas before

continued

Sup
R ← → L
Inf

Ascending
cervical

Inferior laryngeal

Superficial
cervical

Inferior thyroid

Suprascapular
Costocervical trunk
Deep cervical

Vertebral

Thyrocervical trunk

Superior intercostal

Vagus nerve

Dorsal scapular

Recurrent laryngeal
nerve

Scalenus
anterior

Lateral border
of first rib

Internal thoracic

Anterior
intercostal
1-6

Pericardiacophrenic

Anterior
intercostal
7-9

Musculophrenic

Superior epigastric

Phrenic branch

Subclavian artery

Note: (1) The superficial cervical artery is named 'transverse cervical artery' if it gives origin to the dorsal scapular artery instead of the latter arising separately from the second part of the subclavian artery; (2) phrenic branch of musculophrenic artery anastomoses with inferior phrenic artery

turning medially over its posterior arch.
It then turns anteriorly to pierce the
atlanto-occipital membrane lateral to the
cervicomedullary junction. It pierces the
dura and arachnoid to ascend supero-
medially around the anterior aspect of the
medulla where it joins the artery from the
opposite side at the lower border of the pons
to form the basilar artery. (Other branches,
not illustrated, are spinal, meningeal and
muscular.)

Internal thoracic artery. Arises from the
anterior aspect of the first part of the
subclavian artery and passes inferiorly
behind the brachiocephalic vein and the
phrenic nerve to reach the dome of the
pleura. It then angles medially to lie
posterior to the upper six costal cartilages,
between the internal intercostal and
transversus thoracis muscles. It terminates at
the 6th intercostal space to give the superior
epigastric and musculophrenic arteries.
(Other branches, not illustrated, are
mediastinal, thymic, sternal and perforating
(mammary).)

Inferior thyroid artery. Ascends along the
medial edge of scalenus anterior. Just below
the anterior tubercle of C6 it turns medially
to reach the lower thyroid gland, passing
between vertebral artery and vein
(posteriorly) and carotid sheath and
sympathetic chain (anteriorly). Its terminal
branches are often amongst the recurrent
laryngeal nerve. (Other branches of inferior
thyroid artery, not illustrated, are glandular,
pharyngeal, oesophageal and tracheal.)

Superior intercostal artery. Passes inferiorly,
anterior to the necks of the first two ribs to
provide the posterior intercostal arteries for
the first two intercostal spaces.

I

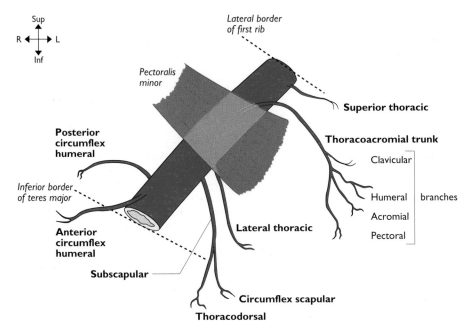

Axillary artery

AXILLARY ARTERY
From: Subclavian art
To: Brachial art

This is the continuation of the subclavian artery. It commences at the lateral border of the 1st rib and ends at the inferior border of teres major to become the brachial artery. It is divided into three parts by pectoralis minor. It is invested in a fascial sheath arising from the prevertebral fascia.

First part is medial to the upper border of pectoralis minor and has one branch. Anterior to it is the clavipectoral fascia, subclavius and the lateral pectoral nerve. The axillary vein is medial whilst posterior to it are the upper part of serratus anterior, the long thoracic nerve, the medial pectoral nerve and the medial cord of the brachial plexus. Lateral to it are the lateral and posterior cords of the brachial plexus.

Second part has pectoralis minor lying anterior to it and has two branches. Medial to it is the axillary vein and medial cord of the brachial plexus. Posterior to it are the posterior cord and subscapularis whilst lateral to it is the lateral cord of the brachial plexus.

Third part extends from the lower border of pectoralis minor to the inferior border of teres major and has three branches. Anterior to it are pectoralis major, the clavipectoral fascia and the median nerve. Medial to it lie the axillary vein and the ulnar nerve. Posterior to it are the radial nerve, teres major, subscapularis and the tendon of latissimus dorsi. On its lateral side lie the musculocutaneous nerve, lateral root (head) of the median nerve, the tendon of biceps in the bicipital groove and coracobrachialis.

Posterior circumflex humeral artery. Passes posteriorly through the quadrangular space with the axillary nerve to supply shoulder joint and surrounding muscles.

Note. Lateral thoracic artery and pectoral branches of the thoraco-acromial trunk are important supply vessels for the breast.

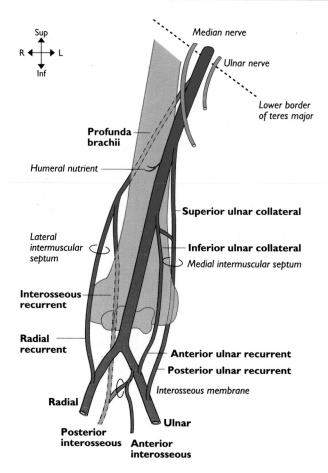

Brachial artery

BRACHIAL ARTERY
From: **Axillary art**
To: **Radial & ulnar arts**

This is the continuation of the axillary artery beginning at the lower margin of the teres major and ending in the cubital fossa at the level of the neck of the radius as the radial and ulnar arteries. At first it lies medial to the humerus then it spirals around to lie anterior to it. It is superficial throughout its course and accompanied by venae commitantes. It is crossed from lateral to medial by the median nerve in the mid arm and by the bicipital aponeurosis in the cubital fossa. Medial to it is the ulnar nerve in the upper arm and, distally, the median nerve. Lateral to it high up are the median and musculo-cutaneous nerves. Coracobrachialis, biceps and its tendon also lie on its lateral side. The artery lies first on the long and then the medial head of triceps, then brachialis in the lower third of the arm.

Arteria profunda brachii. Leaves the posteromedial aspect of the brachial artery just below teres major and passes posteriorly between the long and medial heads of triceps with the radial nerve and into the radial groove before breaking up into its terminal branches.

I

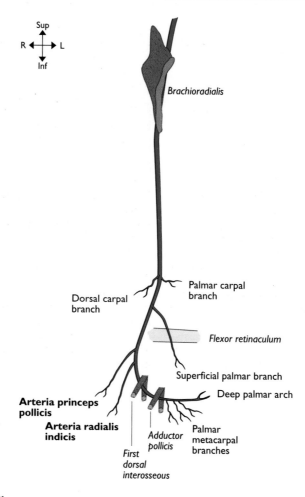

Sup

R ←——→ L

Inf

Brachioradialis

Palmar carpal branch

Dorsal carpal branch

Flexor retinaculum

Superficial palmar branch

Deep palmar arch

Arteria princeps pollicis

Arteria radialis indicis

Adductor pollicis

Palmar metacarpal branches

First dorsal interosseous

Radial artery

RADIAL ARTERY
From: Brachial art in midline of cubital fossa
To: Deep palmar arch in hand

The radial artery arises at the terminal bifurcation of the brachial artery in the cubital fossa at the level of the neck of the radius. It crosses anterior to the biceps tendon to lie initially on supinator. It then passes down the radial side of the forearm lying consecutively on pronator teres, the radial head of flexor digitorum superficialis, flexor pollicis longus and the insertion of pronator quadratus before passing onto the lower end of the radius where its pulse is palpable as it lies lateral to the tendon of flexor carpi radialis. It thus lies deep to brachioradialis and, to a lesser extent, flexor carpi radialis. The superficial branch of the radial nerve lies lateral to it in the forearm. It gives off a palmar carpal branch which contributes to the palmar carpal arch. It then gives off a superficial palmar branch (palmar cutaneous branch) which supplies the thenar muscles before anastomosing with the superficial palmar arch. The radial artery then passes beneath the tendons of abductor pollicis longus and extensor pollicis brevis to enter the anatomical snuff box. It passes across the snuff box on the scaphoid and trapezium and under the tendon of extensor pollicis longus. It gives off a dorsal carpal branch to the dorsal carpal arch which in turn supplies the wrist joint, the dorsal aspects of the metacarpals and the dorsal digital arteries. The radial artery then gives off two named vessels—arteria radialis indicis and princeps pollicis (first palmar metacarpal artery). It next passes down between the two heads of the first dorsal interosseous then between the two heads of adductor pollicis to enter the palm of the hand and form the deep palmar arch. The deep palmar arch lies 1 cm proximal to the superficial palmar arch (ulnar artery). It supplies the palmar metacarpals, gives off a recurrent branch to the palmar carpal arch and three perforating branches which anastomose with the dorsal metacarpal arteries.

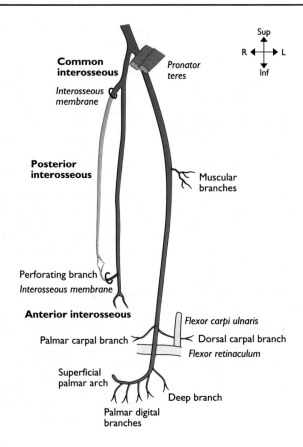

Ulnar artery

ULNAR ARTERY
From: Brachial art
To: Superficial palmar arch in hand

The artery arises as the terminal bifurcation of the brachial artery in the cubital fossa at the level of the neck of the radius. It leaves the fossa deep to the deep head of pronator teres and deep to the fibrous arch of flexor digitorum superficialis just lateral to the median nerve to cross beneath the nerve before running down the ulnar side of the forearm. It lies on flexor digitorum profundus with the ulnar nerve on its medial side. It lies lateral to flexor carpi ulnaris before passing superficial to the flexor retinaculum. The dorsal and palmar carpal arteries contribute, with similarly named arteries from the radial artery, to the dorsal and palmar carpal arches. The ulnar artery then gives off a deep branch to the deep palmar arch before forming the superficial palmar arch at the level of the distal border of the extended thumb. The superficial arch supplies the hypothenar eminence and gives off the palmar digital arteries. At the level of pronator teres the ulnar artery gives off the common interosseous artery which divides into anterior and posterior interosseous arteries.

Anterior interosseous artery. Descends on the anterior surface of the interosseous membrane together with the anterior interosseous branch of the median nerve lying between flexor digitorum profundus medially and flexor pollicis longus laterally. Branches perforate the membrane to supply the extensor muscles. Above pronator quadratus it gives off a small branch which descends deep to the muscle to join the palmar carpal arch, then the anterior interosseous artery itself passes posteriorly through the membrane to anastomose with the posterior interosseous artery which descends to join the dorsal carpal arch.

Posterior interosseous artery. Passes posteriorly above the interosseous membrane and then runs between supinator superficially and abductor pollicis longus deeply with the deep branch of the radial nerve (posterior interosseous nerve) to descend to supply the extensor muscles of the forearm. It anastomoses with the distal branches of the anterior interosseous artery and dorsal carpal arch.

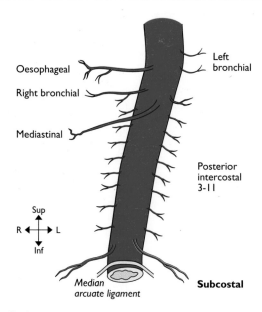

Oesophageal

Left bronchial

Right bronchial

Mediastinal

Posterior intercostal 3-11

Sup

R ← → L

Inf

Median arcuate ligament

Subcostal

Thoracic (descending) aorta

THORACIC (DESCENDING) AORTA
From: Arch of aorta
To: Abdominal aorta

This arises as the continuation of the arch of the aorta commencing to the left of the body of T4 and ends as it passes into the abdomen at T12. It grooves the left side of the bodies of T4–T6 vertebrae then it inclines medially to lie in the midline over the lower thoracic vertebrae. It passes out of the thorax at T12 posterior to the median arcuate ligament of the diaphragm to become the abdominal aorta. Lying anterior to it from above down are the hilum of the left lung (particularly the left main bronchus), pericardium, left atrium, oesophagus and diaphragm. Posterior lie the necks of the ribs of T5–T6 and the sympathetic chain at that level, the vertebral bodies and hemiazygos veins. To its right lie the right pleura and lung and thoracic duct. The oesophagus and its surrounding plexus of nerves is initially to its right but lower down it crosses the aorta to lie anterior then slightly to the left. To its left are the left pleura and lung. (Other branch, not illustrated, is pericardial.)

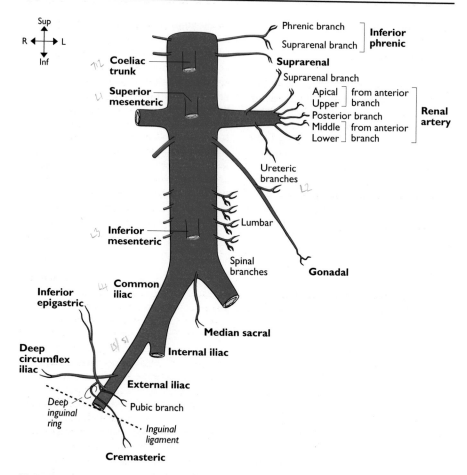

Abdominal aorta & external iliac artery

ABDOMINAL AORTA
From: Thoracic aorta
To: Common iliac arts

This main artery arises as the continuation of the thoracic aorta as it passes, in the midline, posterior to the median arcuate ligament of the diaphragm at T12 and it ends slightly to the left of the midline at L4 where it terminates as the left and right common iliac arteries. Anterior to it, from above downwards, are the coeliac trunk and its branches, the coeliac plexus, lesser sac, superior mesenteric artery, left renal vein, body of pancreas, commencement of each gonadal artery, fourth part of the duodenum, posterior parietal peritoneum, attachment of the mesentery and inferior mesenteric artery. Posterior to it are the lumbar arteries and left lumbar veins, anterior longitudinal ligament and vertebral bodies with their intervertebral discs. To its right are the cisterna chyli, thoracic duct, azygos vein, right crus of diaphragm and inferior vena cava. To its left are the left crus of diaphragm, left coeliac ganglion, the duodenojejunal flexure (upper border of L2), sympathetic trunk and inferior mesenteric vessels. On both sides the phrenic, suprarenal and renal vessels are lateral whilst distal to the bifurcation of the abdominal aorta is the median sacral artery.

Common iliac arteries. These commence at the bifurcation of the abdominal aorta just to the left of the midline at L4 and pass inferolaterally to the level between L5 and S1 vertebrae where they bifurcate anterior to the sacro-iliac joint to give the external and internal iliac arteries. Anterior to each vessel are sympathetic contributions to the superior hypogastric plexus, the ureter (near the terminal bifurcation of the vessel), peritoneum and small bowel. In addition on the left side the superior rectal artery lies anterior. Posterior to each vessel are the sympathetic trunk, obturator nerve, lumbosacral trunk, iliolumbar artery and the bodies of L4 and L5 with the disc between them. In addition posteriorly on the right side are the terminal portions of the common iliac veins and the commencement of the inferior vena cava. The left common iliac vein lies posteromedial to the left common iliac artery. Psoas major lies lateral to each vessel.

Gonadal artery. Descends passing obliquely inferiorly on the posterior abdominal wall to the level of the external iliac artery. The testicular arteries pass around the lower border of the false pelvis to enter the inguinal canal through the deep ring to form part of the spermatic cord. The ovarian vessels descend over the external iliac vessels into the infundibulopelvic fold to supply the ovary via the broad ligament. The common relations of the arteries in both sexes are: left, posterior—psoas, genitofemoral nerve, ureter and external iliac artery; left, anterior—inferior mesenteric vein, left colic artery and sigmoid mesentery; right, posterior—inferior vena cava, psoas, genitofemoral nerve, ureter and external iliac artery; right, anterior—third part of the duodenum, right colic artery and ileal mesentery.

EXTERNAL ILIAC ARTERY
From: Common iliac art
To: Femoral art

The external iliac artery descends laterally from the common iliac artery to pass under the inguinal ligament at the mid inguinal point (half way between the anterior superior iliac spine and symphysis pubis) where it becomes the femoral artery. Posterior and lateral to it is the medial border of psoas major whilst the femoral vein comes to lie medially. Anteromedially it is covered by peritoneum on which lies small bowel with sigmoid colon additionally on the left. It is crossed at its origin by the ureter and then by the gonadal vessels, genital branch of the genitofemoral nerve, deep circumflex iliac vein and vas deferens or round ligament.

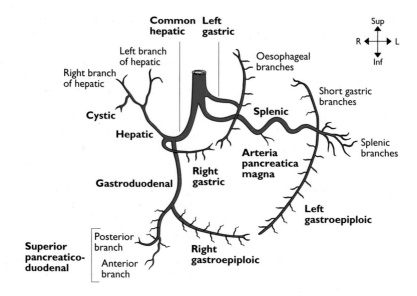

Coeliac trunk

COELIAC TRUNK

From: Abdominal aorta at lower border of
   T12
To: Terminal brs—left gastric, splenic &
   common hepatic arts

The coeliac trunk (axis) arises from the
anterior aspect of the abdominal aorta at the
level of the lower border of T12 and after
1 cm divides into its three terminal branches.

Left gastric artery. Passes superolaterally on
the posterior wall of the lesser sac to reach
the apex of this structure at the cardio-
oesophageal junction where it divides into
oesophageal branches to supply the lower
third of the oesophagus through the
oesophageal opening in the diaphragm.
Its terminal gastric branches run inferiorly
along the upper portion of the lesser curve of
the stomach to anastomose with the right
gastric artery.

Splenic artery. Passes laterally to the left,
angled slightly superiorly, running in the
posterior wall of the lesser sac. Its course
is markedly tortuous as it runs along the
superior border of the pancreas, passing
anterior to the left crus of the diaphragm,
the upper pole of the left kidney and the
left suprarenal gland before entering the
lienorenal ligament to reach the splenic
hilum.

Common hepatic artery. Runs
inferolaterally to the right in the posterior
wall of the lesser sac towards the first part
of the duodenum where it gives off first the
gastroduodenal and then right gastric
arteries. It then curves anteriorly as the
hepatic artery to pass into the peritoneal
reflection which forms the inferior margin of
the opening of the lesser sac. It approaches
the portal vein from its left side and then
comes to lie anterior to it, with the bile duct
on its right, as it ascends in the free border of
the lesser omentum (anterior margin of the
foramen of Winslow or epiploic foramen)
before terminating at the porta hepatis as the
right and left hepatic branches.

Gastroduodenal artery. Descends directly
behind the first part of the duodenum to the
left of the bile duct and divides at the upper
border of the pancreas into terminal
branches.

Right gastric artery. Arises from the hepatic
artery as it enters the lesser omentum and
passes along the lesser curve of the stomach
to anastomose with the left gastric artery.

Superior mesenteric artery

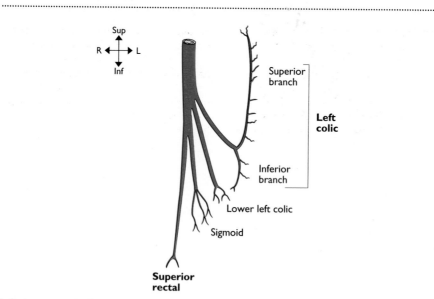

Inferior mesenteric artery

SUPERIOR MESENTERIC ARTERY
From: Abdominal aorta
To: Terminal brs

The superior mesenteric artery arises from the anterior surface of the abdominal aorta at the level of L1. It passes inferiorly over the left renal vein with the splenic vein and body of pancreas anterior to it. It next lies on the uncinate process of the pancreas and the junction of the third and fourth parts of the duodenum from where it passes obliquely and to the right into the mesentery of the small bowel before giving off its terminal branches. The superior mesenteric vein is on its right whilst posterior to the terminal branches are the inferior vena cava, the right ureter and psoas major. The superior mesenteric plexus of nerves surrounds the artery. It supplies bowel from the mid second part of the duodenum, jejunum, ileum, ascending and right two-thirds of transverse colon.

Inferior pancreaticoduodenal artery. Leaves the superior mesenteric artery as it begins to cross the duodenum and divides into an anterior and posterior branch. The anterior branch passes to the right to anastomose with the anterior superior pancreatico-duodenal artery anterior to the head of the pancreas. The posterior branch passes also to the right but posterior to the head of the pancreas to anastomose with the posterior superior pancreaticoduodenal artery.

Middle colic artery. Note that this artery arises early from the superior mesenteric artery to supply the transverse colon. This is logical as the right colic would otherwise need to be excessively long.

Ileocolic artery. Passes obliquely inferiorly to the right in the root of the mesentery where it passes anterior to the right ureter and right gonadal vessels to reach the caecum where it divides into its terminal branches.

INFERIOR MESENTERIC ARTERY
From: Abdominal aorta
To: Terminal brs

This artery arises from the anterior surface of the abdominal aorta at the level of L3 posterior to the third and fourth part of the duodenum. It passes inferiorly and to the left crossing the left common iliac artery medial to the left ureter. The inferior mesenteric vein lies on its left (lateral) side. It divides into its terminal branches in the descending mesocolon. It supplies the left third of the transverse colon, the descending and sigmoid colon and the rectum to the dentate line of the anus.

Internal iliac artery

Femoral artery

INTERNAL ILIAC ARTERY
From: Common iliac art
To: Terminal brs

The artery commences at the level of the disc between L5 and S1 and passes posteriorly into the pelvis for 4 cm before forming anterior and posterior divisions which break up into their terminal branches. Anterior lie the ureter and fallopian tube and ovary in the female. Posterior are the internal iliac vein, lumbosacral trunk and sacro-iliac joint. On the lateral side are the external iliac artery and vein, obturator nerve and psoas major. The parietal peritoneum and small bowel lie medially.

Internal pudendal artery. Arises from the anterior division of the internal iliac artery and descends on the lateral wall of the pelvis towards the greater sciatic foramen. It leaves the pelvis via this foramen, inferior to piriformis, before passing over the tip of the ischial spine to enter the ischio-anal fossa via the lesser sciatic foramen. In runs on the lateral wall of the ischio-anal fossa on obturator internus in the pudendal (Alcock's) canal. It passes into the deep perineal pouch where it gives off its terminal branches. (Other branches of the perineal branch, not illustrated, are transverse perineal and posterior scrotal.)

Note: In the female the vaginal artery is equivalent to the inferior vesical artery in the male, and the uterine artery is equivalent to the middle rectal artery. The round ligament is supplied by the uterine artery whilst the vas deferens is usually supplied by the inferior vesical or less often by the superior vesical artery.

FEMORAL ARTERY
From: External iliac art
To: Popliteal art

This is the continuation of the external iliac artery and commences posterior to the inguinal ligament at the mid-inguinal point (half way between the anterior superior iliac spine and the symphysis pubis). It ends as it passes through the adductor hiatus in adductor magnus to become the popliteal artery. It emerges from under the inguinal ligament with the femoral vein medial to it, both within the femoral sheath. Lateral to it and outside the femoral sheath is the femoral nerve. It lies on the tendon of psoas major and is separated from pectineus and adductor longus by the femoral vein which comes to lie progressively more posterior to the artery within the femoral triangle. As the femoral artery enters the adductor canal it lies on adductor longus then adductor magnus. It is covered initially only by deep fascia then by sartorius; the saphenous nerve passes anteriorly from lateral to medial. Anterolateral to the artery is vastus medialis.

Profunda femoris is the main branch of the femoral artery which is given off posterolaterally just below the femoral sheath 3.5 cm below the inguinal ligament. It runs posteriorly between pectineus and adductor longus to pass into the deep thigh where it provides the deep structures and the posterior and medial compartments with their main arterial supply. Perforating and descending branches anastomose with the genicular branches of the popliteal artery.

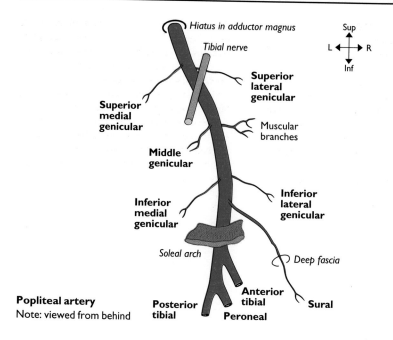

Popliteal artery
Note: viewed from behind

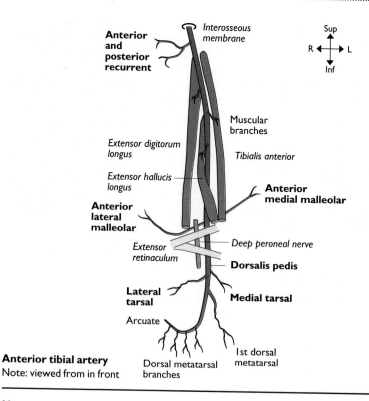

Anterior tibial artery
Note: viewed from in front

POPLITEAL ARTERY
From: Femoral art
To: Ant & post tibial arts

This artery commences as the continuation of the femoral artery as the latter passes through the hiatus in adductor magnus and ends as it passes under the fibrous arch of soleus where it immediately divides into anterior and posterior tibial arteries. The popliteal artery extends from a hand's breadth above the knee and to the same distance below it. It enters the popliteal fossa medial to the femur and becomes the deepest structure, lying with only fat between it and the popliteal surface of the femur. Lower down it lies on the capsule of the knee joint and then on popliteus. Biceps femoris is lateral to it and semimembranosus medial. Lower down it lies between the two heads of gastrocnemius. It is crossed laterally to medially by the tibial nerve and the popliteal vein with the vein always between the artery and nerve.

ANTERIOR TIBIAL ARTERY
From: Popliteal art
To: Dorsalis pedis art

This artery commences at the bifurcation of the popliteal artery just under the fibrous arch of soleus, at the distal border of popliteus. It supplies the structures in the extensor compartment of the lower leg. It passes anteriorly between the heads of tibialis posterior to pass above the upper border of the interosseous membrane, medial to the neck of the fibula accompanied by its venae commitantes. It descends on the interosseous membrane and crosses the lower tibia at the ankle joint, mid way between the malleoli and there becomes the dorsalis pedis artery. Initially it lies between tibialis anterior (medially) and extensor digitorum longus (laterally), then between tibialis anterior and extensor hallucis longus. At the ankle it is crossed anteriorly by the extensor retinacula and also from lateral to medial by the tendon of extensor hallucis longus. The deep peroneal nerve is initially lateral to the artery high up in the extensor compartment but passes anterior to it half way down the leg, becoming lateral to it again under the extensor retinaculum. The anterior tibial veins run in close association with the artery throughout.

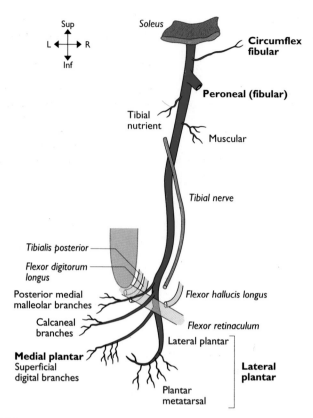

Sup

L ←┼→ R

Inf

Soleus

Circumflex fibular

Peroneal (fibular)

Tibial nutrient

Muscular

Tibial nerve

Tibialis posterior

Flexor digitorum longus

Posterior medial malleolar branches

Flexor hallucis longus

Calcaneal branches

Flexor retinaculum

Lateral plantar

Medial plantar
Superficial digital branches

Lateral plantar

Plantar metatarsal

Posterior tibial artery
Note: viewed from behind

POSTERIOR TIBIAL ARTERY
From: Popliteal art
To: Med & lat plantar arts

This artery arises at the bifurcation of the popliteal artery just under the fibrous arch of soleus, at the lower border of popliteus, and ends by bifurcating into the medial and lateral plantar arteries deep to abductor hallucis. It supplies structures in the posterior compartment of the lower leg. It is accompanied by venae commitantes and lies from above downwards on tibialis posterior, flexor digitorum longus, the tibia and the ankle joint. It lies deep to gastrocnemius, soleus, the flexor retinaculum and abductor hallucis. Posterior to the medial malleolus it lies between the tendon of flexor digitorum longus and the tibial nerve which crosses posterior to the artery mid way down the calf from the medial side to become postero-lateral. (Other branch, not illustrated, is a communicating branch to peroneal (fibular) artery.)

I

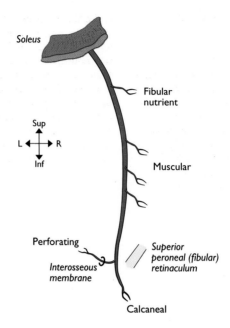

Peroneal (fibular) artery

PERONEAL (FIBULAR) ARTERY
From: Post tibial art
To: Terminal brs

This is a branch of the posterior tibial artery arising 2.5 cm below its origin under soleus. It supplies structures in the lateral compartment of the lower leg. Due to the proximity of origin of the three terminal branches of the popliteal artery this point of origin is commonly referred to as the 'popliteal trifurcation'. It passes inferolaterally to reach and run along the medial crest of the fibula between tibialis posterior and flexor hallucis longus to divide into its terminal branches at the level of the inferior tibiofibular joint and the superior peroneal (fibular) retinaculum. Thus, although it supplies the peroneal compartment by branches that pass laterally, the main peroneal artery itself remains in the posterior compartment. Above, it is covered by soleus and deep fascia whilst in the lower leg flexor hallucis longus crosses it from lateral to medial.

I

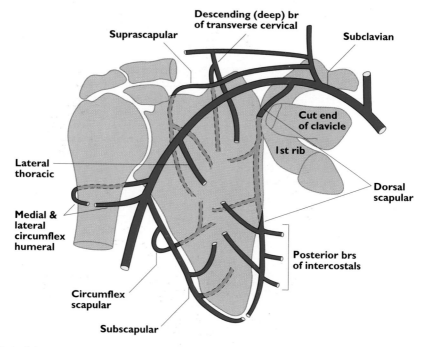

Suprascapular

**Descending (deep) br
of transverse cervical**

Subclavian

**Cut end
of clavicle**

1st rib

**Lateral
thoracic**

**Dorsal
scapular**

**Medial &
lateral
circumflex
humeral**

**Posterior brs
of intercostals**

**Circumflex
scapular**

Subscapular

Arterial anastomoses around scapula

Arterial anastomoses around hip

2: VEINS

2

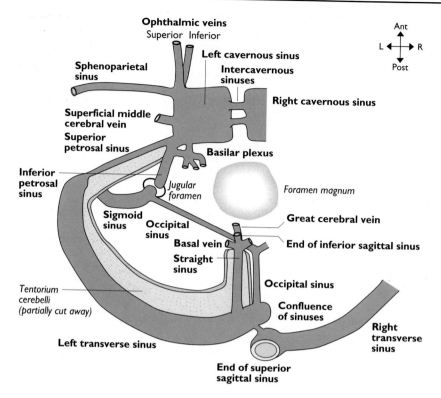

Ophthalmic veins
Superior Inferior
Left cavernous sinus
Sphenoparietal sinus
Intercavernous sinuses
Right cavernous sinus
Superficial middle cerebral vein
Superior petrosal sinus
Basilar plexus
Inferior petrosal sinus
Jugular foramen
Foramen magnum
Sigmoid sinus
Occipital sinus
Great cerebral vein
Basal vein
End of inferior sagittal sinus
Straight sinus
Tentorium cerebelli (partially cut away)
Occipital sinus
Confluence of sinuses
Left transverse sinus
Right transverse sinus
End of superior sagittal sinus

Ant
L ← → R
Post

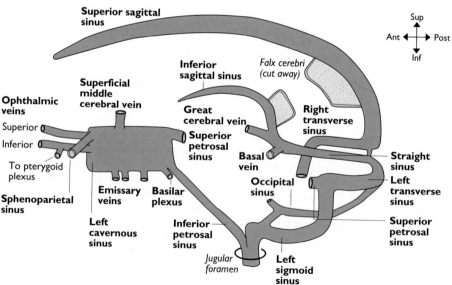

Superior sagittal sinus
Inferior sagittal sinus
Falx cerebri (cut away)
Superficial middle cerebral vein
Ophthalmic veins
Superior
Inferior
Great cerebral vein
Right transverse sinus
Superior petrosal sinus
Basal vein
Straight sinus
To pterygoid plexus
Occipital sinus
Left transverse sinus
Sphenoparietal sinus
Emissary veins
Basilar plexus
Left cavernous sinus
Inferior petrosal sinus
Superior petrosal sinus
Jugular foramen
Left sigmoid sinus

Sup
Ant ← → Post
Inf

Intracranial sinuses & veins

2

INTRACRANIAL SINUSES & VEINS
From: Cerebrum, cerebellum & diploe of
 the skull
To: Internal jugular V

The cerebrum, cerebellum and bones of the
skull are drained by the external, internal
and meningeal veins to the sinuses. The
sinuses lie between the endosteal and
meningeal layers of the dura mater, either as
an endothelial lined space in its free edge
(inferior sagittal and straight sinuses), or a
similarly lined space where the dura is
reflected over the bone of the inner surface
of the skull. They are characteristically thin
walled, contain no valves and communicate
freely with each other.

Superior sagittal sinus. Lies in the superior
margin of the falx cerebri draining the
arachnoid granulations as it does so. It
commences at the foramen caecum and,
posteriorly, usually drains as a continuation
into the right transverse sinus. It frequently
connects at its termination with the left
transverse sinus.

Inferior sagittal sinus. Runs in the inferior
free margin of the falx cerebri draining
medial cortical veins as it does so, and
terminates by fusing with the great cerebral
vein of Galen and right and left basal veins to
form the straight sinus.

Straight sinus. Runs in the junction of the
falx cerebri and tentorium cerebelli for a
short distance before terminating in its
continuation—the left transverse sinus.

Transverse (lateral) sinus. Runs in the lateral
border of the tentorium cerebelli grooving
the occipital and squamous temporal bones,
to terminate in the sigmoid sinus just as it
receives the superior petrosal sinus from the
cavernous sinus on each side.

Sigmoid sinus. Deeply grooves the temporal
bone as it passes inferomedially into the
posterior compartment of the jugular

foramen at the inferior margin of which it
unites with the inferior petrosal sinus to
form the internal jugular vein.

Cavernous sinus. Lies on the lateral wall of
the body of the sphenoid bone and is a lateral
relation of the sella turcica, the pituitary
gland and the sphenoidal air sinus. It lies
medial to the medial gyrus of the temporal
lobe. Lying in it is the internal carotid artery
(carotid syphon) with the abducent nerve
(VI) on its lateral surface and lying on its
lateral wall are nerves (from above down):
oculomotor (III), trochlear (IV), ophthalmic
(Va) and maxillary (Vb) divisions of the
trigeminal. It has a sponge-like reticular
structure and its connections, particularly
those with the other major sinuses (as shown
opposite), frequently provide both supply to,
and drainage from, the sinus. There are two
intercavernous sinuses connecting the
cavernous sinuses to each other.

Occipital sinus. Begins at the foramen
magnum and ascends to end in the
confluence of sinuses.

Confluence of sinuses is at the lowest,
posterior end of the superior sagittal sinus at
the point that it turns, usually to the right, to
become the transverse sinus. It connects with
the straight, occipital and opposite transverse
sinuses.

Sphenoparietal sinus. Runs along the lesser
wing of the sphenoid bone and drains into
the cavernous sinus.

Superior petrosal sinus. Runs along the
petrous temporal bone where the edge of
the tentorium cerebelli attaches and hence
connects the cavernous and transverse
sinuses.

Inferior petrosal sinus. Runs inferiorly to
connect the cavernous sinus to the internal
jugular vein. It exits the skull through the
anterior compartment of the jugular
foramen with the glossopharyngeal nerve.

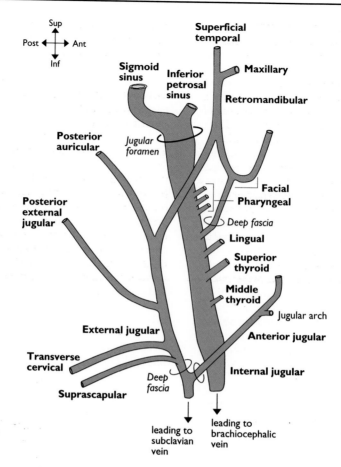

Internal & external jugular veins

INTERNAL JUGULAR VEIN
From: Sigmoid & inf petrosal sinuses
To: Brachiocephalic Vs

It runs almost vertically downwards within the carotid sheath although its covering is thin and readily stretched. Its relationship to the internal carotid artery is as follows: posterior to the artery at the level of C2, posterolateral at C3 and lateral at C4, the vagus nerve (X) lies between the two throughout. Outside the sheath it is surrounded by deep cervical lymph nodes and it lies on (from above down): the lateral mass of the atlas (C1), prevertebral fascia, scalenus medius, scalenus anterior and the dome of the cervical pleura. It is crossed at its origin by the spinal root of the accessory nerve, the lower root of the ansa cervicalis in its middle third and is overlaid by sternocleidomastoid and the tendon of omohyoid in its lower third.

EXTERNAL JUGULAR VEIN
From: Various brs
To: Subclavian V

It arises from the junction of the posterior auricular vein and the posterior division of the retromandibular vein and drains into the subclavian vein. The external jugular system lies within the superficial tissues of the neck (as does the anterior jugular system). The external and anterior jugular veins pierce the deep fascia of the neck, usually posterior to the clavicular head of sternocleidomastoid to fuse before draining into the subclavian vein.

2

Superior vena cava & azygos veins

Note: (1) Accessory hemiazygos crosses to azygos at T7 and hemiazygos at T8—each crosses behind thoracic aorta, oesophagus and thoracic duct; (2) left bronchial vein may enter accessory hemiazygos. *= oesophageal and mediastinal veins, IVC = inferior vena cava, SVC = superior vena cava

SUPERIOR VENA CAVA
From: Brachiocephalic Vs
To: Right atrium

It is formed posterior to the right first costal cartilage and passes posterior to the right sternal border where it is a close posterior relation of the right internal thoracic vessels and sternal periosteum and is occasionally overlaid by the anterior segment of the right upper lobe of the lung. It lies anterolateral to the trachea and upper right lung hilum with the right phrenic nerve applied to its right lateral surface. It receives the azygos vein into its posterior surface at the level of T4. It enters the superior surface of the right atrium without any valvular mechanism guarding its orifice.

Left brachiocephalic vein. Formed posterior to the left sternoclavicular joint and anterior to the cervical pleura. It passes obliquely downwards to the right, posterior to the manubrium, separated from it only by the thymus gland or its remnant. It lies anterior to the left common carotid and brachiocephalic arteries and crosses the upper anterior aortic arch. Unlike the right superior intercostal vein (see below) the left superior intercostal vein drains into the left brachiocephalic vein. Other tributaries (not shown) are thymic and pericardial veins.

Right brachiocephalic vein. Formed posterior to the right sternoclavicular joint and passes directly inferiorly behind the right side of the manubrium, anterolateral to the trachea and anteromedial to the pleura over the upper lobe of the lung.

AZYGOS VEINS
From: Inf vena cava/ascending lumbar Vs
To: Sup vena cava

The azygos veins drain the upper lumbar region and the thoracic wall. There is a single system on the right whilst on the left there are two—the hemiazygos and accessory hemiazygos that drain over into the azygos separately.

Azygos vein. Arises at the approximate level of the right renal vein either as a posterior tributary of the inferior vena cava or as a confluence of the right ascending lumbar and right subcostal vein. It passes through the aortic opening of the diaphragm under the right crus at the level of T12 vertebra and ascends on the right side of the vertebral bodies behind the oesophagus. It turns anteriorly to pass over the hilum of the right lung, lateral to the oesophagus, trachea and right vagus, to enter the superior vena cava at the level of T4. Its tributaries are the lower eight right posterior intercostal veins, the right superior intercostal vein (draining the 2nd, 3rd and 4th right intercostal veins), bronchial and oesophageal veins and, from the left side, the two hemiazygos veins.

Hemiazygos vein. Arises from the confluence of the left ascending lumbar vein, the left subcostal vein and often a tributary from the left renal vein. It ascends through the aortic opening of the diaphragm and onto the left side of the thoracic vertebra to the level of T9 from where it crosses posterior to the aorta, oesophagus and thoracic duct to enter the azygos vein at T8. It drains the four lower left posterior intercostal veins (9–12th).

Accessory hemiazygos vein. Drains the 5–8th left posterior intercostal veins and runs inferiorly on the left side of the vertebral bodies to T8 where it crosses similarly to the hemiazygos vein to enter the azygos vein at T7. It also receives tributaries from the bronchial and mid-oesophageal veins.

Note: The anterior intercostal veins drain to the musculophrenic and internal thoracic veins.

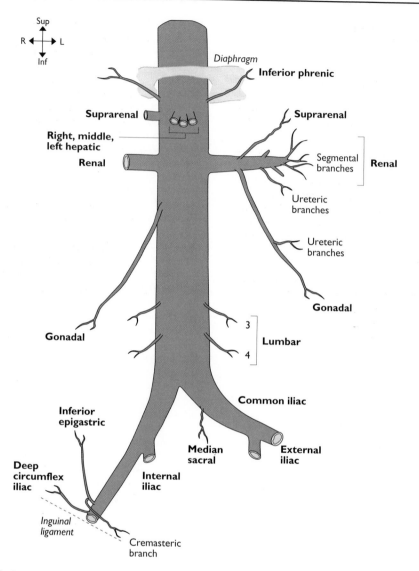

Sup

R ←→ L

Inf

Diaphragm

Inferior phrenic

Suprarenal

Suprarenal

Right, middle, left hepatic

Segmental branches

Renal

Renal

Ureteric branches

Ureteric branches

Gonadal

Gonadal

3

4

Lumbar

Common iliac

Inferior epigastric

External iliac

Median sacral

Deep circumflex iliac

Internal iliac

Inguinal ligament

Cremasteric branch

Inferior vena cava

INFERIOR VENA CAVA
From: Common iliac Vs
To: Right atrium

It arises as the fusion of the common iliac veins anterolateral to the L5 vertebral body lying posterior to the right common iliac artery. It ascends, initially posterolateral to, then lateral to the aorta and lies anterolateral to the right of the bodies of L5–L1. It lies on (from below up): right lumbar arteries, right renal artery, right sympathetic chain, right suprarenal gland, right crus of the diaphragm and right inferior phrenic artery. It is crossed by (from below up): the root of the ileal mesentery, the third part of the duodenum, the head of the pancreas, the bile duct, the portal vein, the first part of the duodenum, the posterior abdominal peritoneum and the bare area of the liver.

It is hugged closely on its right side by the right suprarenal gland and forms the posterior wall of the epiploic foramen of Winslow below this. After passing through the caval orifice in the central tendon of the diaphragm (T8) with the right phrenic nerve lateral to it, it almost immediately enters the pericardium and then the inferior aspect of the right atrium. The vein possesses a 'valve-like' flap guarding the medial portion of its orifice.

Lumbar veins. Drain somewhat inconsistently but usually the 3rd and 4th drain directly into the inferior vena cava whilst above this level they drain into the ascending lumbar veins and hence to the azygos and hemiazygos systems. There are, however, usually connections of the 3rd and 4th lumbar veins with the ascending lumbar veins.

2

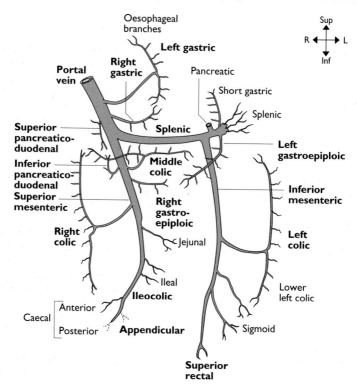

Portal vein

PORTAL VEIN
From: **Sup mesenteric & splenic Vs**
To: **Porta hepatis**

The vein is formed from the union of the superior mesenteric and splenic veins at the level of the disc between L1 and L2 just at the right of the midline. At its formation it lies posterior to the neck of the pancreas and anterior to the inferior vena cava. It runs superiorly inclining slightly to the right, lying posterior to the first part of the duodenum and anterior to the inferior vena cava. The bile duct comes to lie anterolateral to it from the right and the hepatic artery comes to lie anteromedial to it from the left. Ascending in the free border of the lesser omentum it continues to lie posterior to these two structures and forms the anterior margin of the aditus to the lesser sac (foramen of Winslow). It divides into terminal right and left branches as it enters the porta hepatis.

Portosystemic anastomoses
1 Lower end of oesophagus. The veins from the lower third of the oesophagus drain downwards to the left gastric vein (portal) and, above this level, oesophageal veins drain to the azygos and hemiazygos systems (systemic).
2 Upper end of anal canal. At the anal columns in the upper half of the anal canal there is a venous watershed between the drainage above by the superior rectal veins (portal via inferior mesenteric vein) and drainage below by the inferior and middle rectal veins (systemic via the pudendal and internal iliac veins).
3 Bare area of liver. Where the bare area of the liver lies in contact with the diaphragm there is a watershed of venous drainage between the hepatic veins (portal) and the inferior phrenic veins (systemic).
4 Periumbilical. The ligamentum teres represents a venous watershed in that its inner portion is drained into the portal system (via the left branch of the portal vein) whilst its outer portion is drained into the systemic system (indirectly via the great saphenous and axillary veins).
5 Retroperitoneal. Branches of the left and right colic and splenic veins (portal) may meet branches of the lumbar veins (systemic via inferior vena cava and azygos systems) in the retroperitoneal area.

2

2

3: LYMPHATICS

Note: Deep lymphatics follow arteries and
superficial ones follow veins.

3

3

Right jugular lymph trunk

Right subclavian lymph trunk

Inferior cervical ganglion

Left jugular lymph trunk

Left subclavian lymph trunk

Scalenus anterior

Right bronchomediastinal lymph trunk

Upper left intercostal and mediastinal lymph trunk

Descending thoracic aorta

Left and right descending thoracic lymph trunks

Right crus of diaphragm

Cisterna chyli (confluence of lymph trunks)

T12

Right and left lumbar and intestinal lymph trunks

Sup

R ← → L

Inf

Thoracic & right lymphatic ducts

THORACIC & RIGHT LYMPHATIC DUCTS
From: Cisterna chyli
To: Left subclavian V

Thoracic duct
Receives:
- Left jugular trunk
- Left subclavian trunk
- Cisterna chyli
- Most thoracic lymphatics (except right upper thorax)

Drains:
- All body tissue below the diaphragm
- Left arm
- Left head and neck
- Left thorax
- Lower right thorax

It originates from the upper cisterna chyli on the right anterolateral side of the body of T12, lying lateral to the abdominal aorta. It passes posterior to the right crus of the diaphragm and ascends on the right posterior intercostal arteries with the aorta on its left and the azygos vein on its right. It slopes to the left in the mid thorax crossing the vertebral column posterior to the oesophagus at the level of T5. It continues superiorly to the left of the vertebral column, posterolateral to the oesophagus, posteromedial to the upper mediastinal pleura and posterior to the initial part of the left subclavian artery. It then passes anterior to the inferior cervical (stellate) ganglion before arching anteriorly over the left vertebral and left subclavian arteries and the dome of the pleura to lie along the medial edge of scalenus anterior before reaching the posterosuperior aspect of the left subclavian vein as the latter joins the left internal jugular vein.

Right lymphatic duct
Receives:
- Right subclavian trunk
- Right jugular trunk
- Right bronchomediastinal trunk (right upper thorax)

Drains:
- Right head and neck
- Right arm
- Right upper thorax

The three trunks usually drain separately but the first two often join to give a right lymphatic duct which ends in the right subclavian vein. In which case it has a very short course from its formation anterior to scalenus anterior, passing over the dome of the cervical pleura to reach the right subclavian vein as the latter joins with the right internal jugular vein.

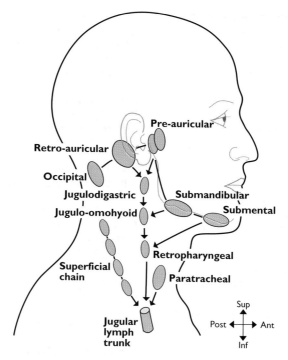

Lymph glands — head & neck

LYMPH GLANDS—HEAD & NECK

Circular nodal chain
Submental (bilateral)
    Anterior tongue
    Floor of mouth
    Lower incisor and canine teeth
    Lower lip
    Skin of anterior chin
Submandibular
    Upper lip
    Cheek
    Nose
    Forehead and anterior scalp
    Middle tongue
    Lower molar and premolar teeth
    All upper teeth
    Sublingual gland
    Submandibular gland
    Anterior half of nasal cavity and nasal
      sinuses
Deep and superficial pre-auricular (parotid)
    Middle scalp
    Skin of temple
    Pinna
    Parotid gland
    Posterior orbit

Retro-auricular (mastoid)
    Pinna
    Posterior scalp
Occipital
    Posterior scalp

Deep cervical chain
Jugulodigastric
    Palatine tonsil
    Upper pharynx
    Posterior tongue
Jugulo-omohyoid
    Posterior half of nasal cavity and nasal
      sinuses
    Palate (hard and soft)
Retropharyngeal
    Pharynx
Paratracheal
    Hypopharynx
    Larynx
    Trachea
    Thyroid
    Parathyroids

Superficial cervical chain
Skin of neck

3

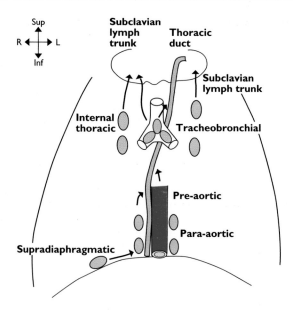

Lymph glands—thorax

LYMPH GLANDS—THORAX

Pre-aortic
  Middle third of oesophagus
Supradiaphragmatic
  Diaphragm
  Subphrenic spaces
  Bare area of liver
Tracheobronchial
  Heart and all layers of pericardium
  Lungs and visceral pleura
  Extrapulmonary bronchi
  Trachea
  Thymus (occasionally thyroid isthmus)
Para-aortic
  Thoracic wall
  Parietal pleura
  Anterior abdominal wall
Internal thoracic
  Breast
  Anterior thoracic wall
  Upper abdominal muscles
  Diaphragm

Left and right lower thoracic nodes drain directly to the thoracic duct or via a separate left bronchiomediastinal trunk which joins the thoracic duct in the posterior superior mediastinum. Upper right thoracic nodes drain via the right bronchomediastinal trunk which either drains into the right lymphatic duct or directly into the right subclavian vein.

Note: Normal drainage from breast is to anterior and posterior axillary, infra-clavicular and internal thoracic groups. With pathological blockage from disease the spread can be to opposite side, cervical, peritoneal cavity and liver, and inguinal glands.

3

3

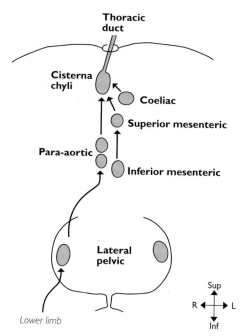

Lymph glands—abdomen

LYMPH GLANDS—ABDOMEN

Coeliac
  Lower third of oesophagus
  Stomach and greater omentum
  First and upper second part of duodenum
  Spleen
  Pancreas
  Liver
  Gallbladder
Superior mesenteric
  Lower second, third and fourth parts of
    duodenum
  Jejunum
  Ileum
  Caecum and appendix
  Ascending colon
  Transverse colon
Inferior mesenteric
  Distal transverse colon
  Descending colon
  Sigmoid colon
  Upper rectum and rectal mucosa to
    dentate line
Para-aortic
  Inferior surface of diaphragm
  Suprarenal gland
  Kidney
  Gonad (plus fallopian tube in female)
  Superior lateral uterus

Ureter
Bare area of liver
Posterior abdominal wall
Lateral pelvic nodes
  Lower rectum and dentate line
  Bladder
  Urethra
  Lower ureter
  Female
    uterus
    cervix
    upper vagina
    clitoris
    labia minora
  Male
    vas deferens
    seminal vesicles
    prostate
    bulk of penis

Endodermal (gut-tube/gut-derived)
structures drain to lymph nodes lying along
their arteries of supply which are named
according to the artery with which they are
associated and are not listed individually.
Their number and exact position are vari-
able. However, the position and drainage of
the highest node groups (listed above) are
constant.

3

3

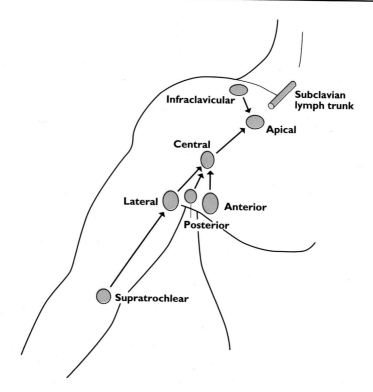

Lymph glands—upper limb

LYMPH GLANDS—UPPER LIMB

Axillary groups
Anterior (pectoral)
  Breast
  Anterior thoracic wall
  Upper anterior abdominal wall
Posterior (subscapular)
  Posterior thoracic wall
  Tail of breast
  Upper posterior abdominal wall
Lateral
  Arm
  Forearm
  Hand

Central
Apical
Supratrochlear
  Skin of anterior forearm and hand
Infraclavicular
  Skin of shoulder
  Skin of lower neck
  Skin of anterior upper thoracic wall
  Breast

A useful mnemonic for the axillary nodes is the word APICAL—(A)nterior, (P)osterior, (I)nfraclavicular, (C)entral, (A)pical, (L)ateral

3

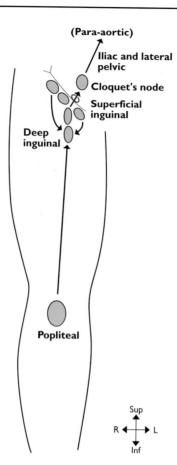

(Para-aortic)

Iliac and lateral pelvic

Cloquet's node

Superficial inguinal

Deep inguinal

Popliteal

Sup

R ← → L

Inf

Lymph glands—lower limb

3

LYMPH GLANDS—LOWER LIMB

Superficial inguinal
   Uterine fundus (via round ligament)
   Skin of penis
   Labia minora/scrotum
   Skin of buttock
   Skin of lower abdominal wall to umbilicus
   Skin of thigh, anterior skin of calf and
     dorsum of foot
   Skin of anterior perineum
Deep inguinal
   Anterior perineum
   Thigh
   Leg
   Foot

Popliteal
   Skin of sole of foot
   Skin of posterior calf

Note: Cloquet's node is the highest node of the lower limb and usually lies just inside the femoral canal beneath the inguinal ligament, medial to the femoral vein and lateral to the lacunar ligament.

Superficial inguinal lymphatics drain via the saphenous opening into the deep inguinal nodes and then via the femoral canal to Cloquet's node and the internal iliac nodes.

4

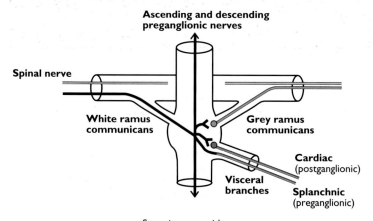

Ascending and descending
preganglionic nerves

Spinal nerve

White ramus
communicans

Grey ramus
communicans

Cardiac
(postganglionic)

Visceral
branches

Splanchnic
(preganglionic)

Somatic nerve with
postganglionic sympathetic

T1

T2

T3

T4

T5

T6

T7

T8

T9

T10

T11

T12

Cardiac branches
(T1-5)
(postganglionic)

Greater splanchnic nerve
(T5-9)
(preganglionic)

Coeliac ganglia
and
suprarenal gland

Aorticorenal ganglia

Lesser splanchnic nerve
(T10-11)
(preganglionic)

Least splanchnic nerve
(T12)
(preganglionic)

Renal plexus

Thoracic sympathetics (T1–12)
Note: All splanchnic nerves synapse in collateral ganglia

4: AUTONOMIC NERVOUS SYSTEM

The autonomic nervous system, as the term implies, is an internal (visceral) adjustment system which is largely controlled automatically but is influenced, to some extent, by somatic activity and the special senses. It controls the activity of the viscera, glands, blood vessels, heart and smooth muscle.

The two parts, working complementarily, are the sympathetic and parasympathetic systems. The sympathetic system is active at times of urgent activity or stress, summarised as the fight, flight and fright response, at which time blood is needed rapidly in muscles and brain and can be diverted there from the skin and gut. There is, therefore, selective vasoconstriction, increase in heart rate and blood pressure together with bronchodilatation, decrease in intestinal peristalsis and closure of sphincters. In addition there are two further activities in the head and neck where the eyes open wide and the pupils dilate. On a less urgent basis somatic nerves to skin carry sympathetic fibres which constantly adjust sweating (sudomotor), blood flow (vasomotor) and hair erection (pilomotor) as a means of heat regulation.

Conversely, parasympathetic activity predominates during periods of quiet activity, rest and during and after feeding when the salivary glands secrete and food is digested. There is maximal intestinal activity and normal production of glandular secretions from mucosa throughout the body. The heart rate is slowed, blood pressure is minimised, the bronchi constricted to lessen the dead space of the airways and the pupils are constricted. An extra task for the parasympathetic is accommodation of the lens for near vision.

The efferent (motor) nerves of both systems are accompanied by general visceral afferent (sensory) fibres which detect visceral distension, excessive smooth muscle contraction, hunger, nausea and sexual excitement. From the heart and lungs sensation is probably in both sympathetic and parasympathetic systems whereas in the abdomen it is predominantly in the sympathetic system. Sensation from pelvic organs of cloacal origin travel with the parasympathetics.

Sympathetic

The following 10 'rules' summarise the general plan for the sympathetics:

1 Sympathetic motor function stimulates: sweating, pilo-erection and vascular constriction in the skin. Throughout the rest of the body it controls vascular calibre and smooth muscle tone, stimulating closure of sphincters (pylorus, internal anal, vesical). It decreases glandular secretion; causes ejaculation, bronchodilatation; and also increases the heart rate.

2 In addition to these it also has two special functions in the head and neck for dilating the pupil and raising the eyelids.

3 Sympathetic outflow from the spinal cord occurs only from preganglionic cell bodies in the lateral horns of T1 to L2. These myelinated preganglionic fibres (shown in black) exit with the somatic motor root from the ventral horn but soon leave the ventral ramus to pass to the ganglia of the sympathetic chain in a white ramus communicans.

4 Although the spinal connections to the sympathetic chain of ganglia are only between T1 and L2, the chain itself extends the whole length of the body with a ganglion at the level of each spinal nerve in the lumbosacral region and three ganglia above T1—superior, middle and inferior cervical ganglia. The inferior cervical ganglion is usually fused with the T1 ganglion and the two together are then termed the stellate ganglion.

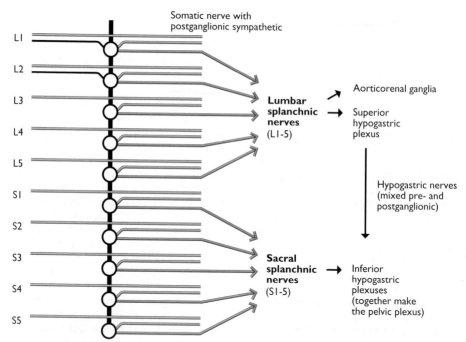

Lumbosacral sympathetics (L1–S5)

Note: L1–2 have white rami communicans. Lumbar and sacral splanchnic nerves are all preganglionic. They synapse in the inferior hypogastric plexus and perhaps some in the superior hypogastric plexus

5 When the preganglionic fibres reach a ganglion of the sympathetic chain they have two alternatives. They can leave that ganglion for distribution, with or without synapsing (see below). Alternatively, they can pass up or down the chain to a higher or lower ganglion before leaving for distribution, with or without synapsing (see below). Thus the upper thoracic sympathetics supply the arm and head and neck regions whilst the lower thoracic and upper lumbar sympathetics supply the lower trunk and leg.

6 In the ganglion from which the sympathetic is destined to leave, the preganglionic fibres always synapse and leave as postganglionic fibres *unless* they are supplying *gut* or *suprarenal gland* in which case they continue as preganglionic fibres.

7 Each ganglion has a somatic (lateral) branch from which unmyelinated postganglionic fibres (shown in green) pass into a grey ramus communicans to reach the somatic nerve at the same level.

8 Each ganglion has a visceral (medial) branch (shown in red) which supplies internal organs, such as the heart, with unmyelinated postganglionic fibres. Note that fibres to the gut and suprarenal gland, in the form of greater, lesser, least, lumbar and sacral splanchnic nerves, are all preganglionic (see 6 above). They synapse in collateral ganglia nearer the organ of distribution (coeliac, renal, inferior hypogastric, etc.) before becoming postganglionic. The medulla of the suprarenal gland can be considered as a ganglion.

9 In addition to the somatic and visceral branches, the three cervical ganglia have vascular (anterior) branches (shown in grey) which are distributed as in the diagram. These vascular branches simply allow a wider distribution of sympathetics to major vessels and into the skull than is possible via somatic or visceral branches. For the special function of pupillary dilatation and eyelid raising these sympathetics are distributed via cranial nerves—ophthalmic division of trigeminal and oculomotor respectively.

10 Sympathetic afferent (sensory) fibres (not shown) from the viscera return along the visceral efferent branches, pass through the ganglia of the sympathetic chain and the white rami communicantes before reaching their cell bodies in the dorsal root ganglia. They enter the spinal cord with the somatic sensory fibres via the dorsal horn. Note that the grey rami communicantes contain postganglionic efferent sympathetics only whilst the white rami communicates contain both preganglionic efferent sympathetic fibres and afferent sympathetic fibres.

Parasympathetic

The following 10 'rules' summarize the general plan for the parasympathetics:

1 Parasympathetic motor function stimulates: glandular secretions, particularly salivary glands and mucous glands throughout the body; peristalsis; opening of sphincters (pylorus and internal anal); penile erection; slowing of the heart; and bronchial constriction.

2 Two special functions in the head and neck are pupillary constriction and accommodation of the lens for near vision.

3 The only parasympathetic outflow in the body is with the cranial nerves III, VII, IX, X and from sacral segments S2,3,4.

4 All myelinated preganglionic efferent fibres (shown in red) that are destined to supply structures in the head and neck emerge from the brain stem with fibres of the relevant cranial nerve (III, VII and IX) and run to specific parasympathetic ganglia where they synapse (see diagram, see p. 78).

5 Each of these peripheral parasympathetic ganglia (ciliary, pterygopalatine, submandibular and otic) have a characteristic pattern of nerve connection in that in addition to the parasympathetic synapse, there is a sensory branch of the trigeminal nerve (V) and vasomotor fibres of the sympathetic both passing straight through the ganglion (see diagram, see p. 79). Beyond the ganglion, the sensory branch of the trigeminal nerve carries the postganglionic, unmyelinated parasympathetic fibres (also shown in red) and the sympathetic fibres to the end organ.

6 Each vagus nerve (X) has two cervical parasympathetic branches that pass down to the heart and then each vagus continues to

4

4

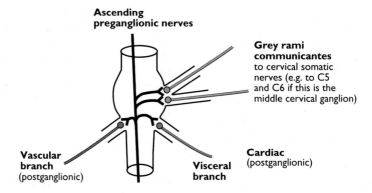

Ascending preganglionic nerves

Grey rami communicantes to cervical somatic nerves (e.g. to C5 and C6 if this is the middle cervical ganglion)

Vascular branch (postganglionic)

Visceral branch

Cardiac (postganglionic)

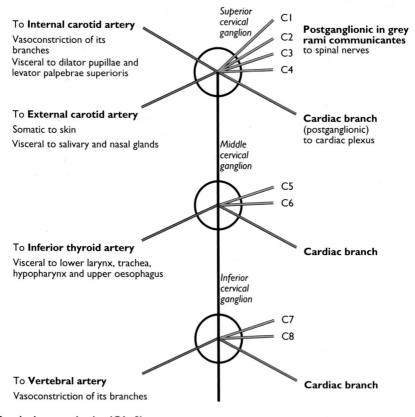

To **Internal carotid artery**

Vasoconstriction of its branches
Visceral to dilator pupillae and levator palpebrae superioris

Superior cervical ganglion

C1
C2
C3
C4

Postganglionic in grey rami communicantes to spinal nerves

To **External carotid artery**

Somatic to skin
Visceral to salivary and nasal glands

Cardiac branch (postganglionic) to cardiac plexus

Middle cervical ganglion

C5
C6

To **Inferior thyroid artery**

Visceral to lower larynx, trachea, hypopharynx and upper oesophagus

Cardiac branch

Inferior cervical ganglion

C7
C8

To **Vertebral artery**
Vasoconstriction of its branches

Cardiac branch

Cervical sympathetics (C1–8)

supply parasympathetic fibres to thoracic and abdominal structures as far as two-thirds along the transverse colon. The preganglionic fibres synapse in peripheral ganglia so that the postganglionic fibres are usually short.

7 The parasympathetic outflow in the sacral region (S2,3,4) arises in the lateral grey horn but emerges via the ventral horn and the fibres constitute a pelvic splanchnic nerve. Each nerve passes to its inferior hypogastric plexus (left and right together making the pelvic plexus) and then to the walls of the pelvic viscera where these preganglionic fibres synapse in small ganglia before distribution. On the left, post-ganglionic fibres pass upwards to the left colon and the left third of the transverse colon via the superior hypogastric plexus and then onto the colic vessels.

8 Although not strictly part of the parasympathetic system, there are afferent (sensory) fibres running with the para-sympathetics. In the vagus (X) there are general visceral afferent fibres from the thorax and abdomen (transmitting pain, visceral distension, etc.) which have their cell bodies in the inferior vagal ganglion and their central connections probably in the nucleus solitarius or dorsal vagal nucleus. For pelvic sensation similar fibres reach sacral segments S2,3,4, with their cell bodies in the dorsal root ganglia before they enter the dorsal horn of the spinal cord.

9 Other sensory fibres running with the parasympathetics are special visceral afferents which detect taste and changes in the baro- and chemoreceptors in the carotid sinus and body respectively.

10 The carotid sinus and body are supplied by both the glossopharyngeal nerve (IX) and the vagus (X) with cell bodies in their respective inferior ganglia. Taste is carried in VII, IX and X. The cell bodies for taste in VII are in the geniculate ganglion, those in IX are in the inferior glossopharyngeal ganglion, whilst those in X are in the inferior vagal ganglion. Central connections are in the nucleus solitarius (see summary table of cranial nerve nuclei and fibres).

4

taste ⟹ CN VII Facial n. (gen=ling.) Chorda Tympani Ant 2/3

Taste + gen' ⟹ CN IX glossopharyngeal n. post 1/3
CN X vagus

4

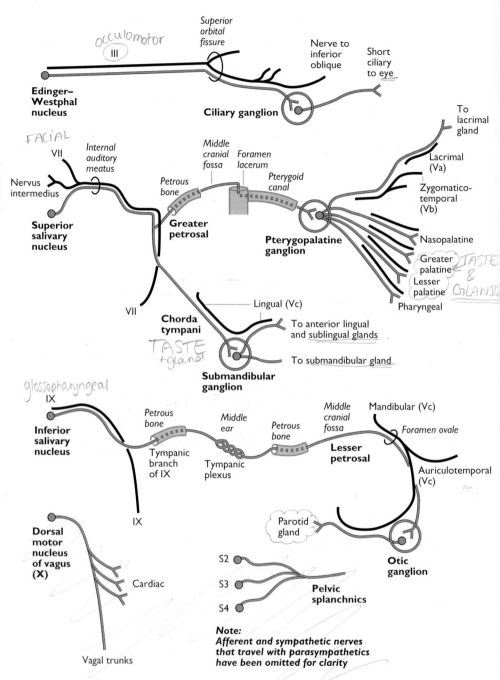

occulomotor

Edinger–Westphal nucleus
Superior orbital fissure
Nerve to inferior oblique
Short ciliary to eye
Ciliary ganglion

FACIAL
VII
Nervus intermedius
Internal auditory meatus
Superior salivary nucleus
Middle cranial fossa
Foramen lacerum
Pterygoid canal
Petrous bone
Greater petrosal
Pterygopalatine ganglion
To lacrimal gland
Lacrimal (Va)
Zygomatico-temporal (Vb)
Nasopalatine
Greater palatine
Lesser palatine
Pharyngeal
TASTE & GLAND

VII
Chorda tympani
Lingual (Vc)
To anterior lingual and sublingual glands
To submandibular gland
TASTE + gland
Submandibular ganglion

glossopharyngeal
IX
Inferior salivary nucleus
Petrous bone
Tympanic branch of IX
Middle ear
Tympanic plexus
Petrous bone
Middle cranial fossa
Lesser petrosal
Mandibular (Vc)
Foramen ovale
Auriculotemporal (Vc)

IX
Dorsal motor nucleus of vagus (X)
Cardiac
Parotid gland
Otic ganglion

S2
S3
S4
Pelvic splanchnics

Vagal trunks

Note:
Afferent and sympathetic nerves that travel with parasympathetics have been omitted for clarity

Parasympathetic system
Note: Afferent nerves and sympathetics that travel with parasympathetics have been omitted for clarity

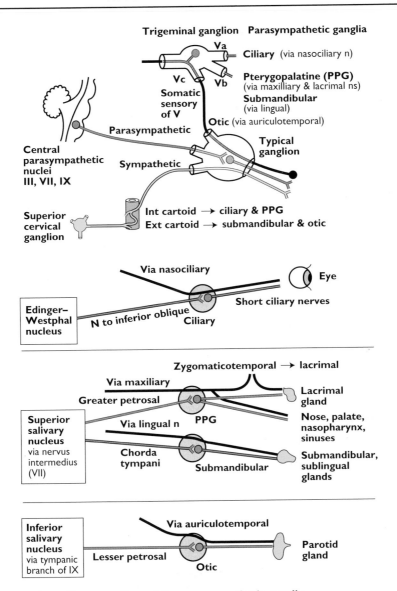

Trigeminal ganglion   Parasympathetic ganglia

Va

Ciliary (via nasociliary n)

Vc   **Vb**

Pterygopalatine (PPG)
(via maxilliary & lacrimal ns)

Somatic
sensory
of V

Submandibular
(via lingual)

Otic (via auriculotemporal)

Parasympathetic

Typical
ganglion

Central
parasympathetic
nuclei
III, VII, IX

Sympathetic

Superior
cervical
ganglion

Int cartoid → **ciliary & PPG**
Ext cartoid → **submandibular & otic**

Via nasociliary

Eye

Edinger–
Westphal
nucleus

N to inferior oblique   Ciliary

Short ciliary nerves

Zygomaticotemporal → **lacrimal**

Via maxillary

Greater petrosal

Lacrimal
gland

Superior
salivary
nucleus
via nervus
intermedius
(VII)

Via lingual n   PPG

Chorda
tympani   **Submandibular**

Nose, palate,
nasopharynx,
sinuses

Submandibular,
sublingual
glands

Inferior
salivary
nucleus
via tympanic
branch of IX

Via auriculotemporal

Lesser petrosal

Otic

Parotid
gland

Typical and specific connections of the parasympathetic ganglia
PPG; pterygopalatine ganglion

4

Pathways for cranial outflow of parasympathetic nerves

Cranial nerve	Central nucleus	Nerve carrying preganglionic fibres	Pathway & foramen	Site of ganglion	Name of ganglion	Nerve carrying postganglionic fibres	Organs supplied
III	Edinger–Westphal (midbrain)	III→ Nerve to inferior oblique	Cavernous sinus→ superior orbital fissure→ orbit	Between optic N & lat rectus in apex of orbit	Ciliary	**Va** Nasociliary & short ciliary	**Ciliary muscle for accommodation. Circular muscle of pupil for constriction**
VII	Superior salivary (pons)	Nervus intermedius →VII→ greater petrosal N→ N of pterygoid canal	Internal acoustic meatus→ middle ear→ middle cranial fossa → pterygoid canal	Pterygopalatine fossa	Pterygopalatine	**Vb** (maxillary branches) **Vb** (infra-orbital → zygomatic → z-temporal) → **Va** (lacrimal)	**Mucosal glands of nose, nasopharynx, sinuses, soft palate** **Lacrimal gland**
VII	Superior salivary (pons)	Nervus intermedius →VII→ chorda tympani → lingual N	Internal acoustic meatus→ middle ear → petrotympanic fissure→ infratemporal fossa	Below lingual N on hyoglossus	Submandibular	**Vc** (lingual)	**Submandibular, sublingual, ant. lingual, mucosal glands on side of tongue**
IX	Inferior salivary (medulla)	IX→ tympanic branch → lesser petrosal N	Middle ear →middle cranial fossa → f. ovale	Below f. ovale on N to tensor tympani & palati	Otic	**Vc** (auriculotemporal)	**Parotid gland**
IX	Inferior salivary (medulla)	Pharyngeal & laryngeal branches	Direct to oropharynx & post third of tongue	In mucosa of oropharynx & post third of tongue			**Mucosal glands of oropharynx, post third of tongue**
X	Dorsal motor (medulla)	X (Vagus)	Cardiac branches from neck→ plexus on oesophagus → abdomen	On target organs			**All viscera of thorax & abdomen → 2/3 across transverse colon (S2,3,4 for rest)**

(handwritten annotation: ant 2/3 tongue + TASTE)

4

4

Cranial nerves
Parasympathetic
Sympathetic
Possible alternative pathway for sympathetic

Edinger–Westphal nucleus
Oculomotor n (III)
Int carotid artery
Trigeminal n
Sup cervical ganglion
Greater petrosal n
Facial n (VII)
Nervus intermedius
Jugular foramen
Glosso-pharyngeal n
Tympanic br of IX
Cavernous sinus
Trigeminal ganglion
Deep petrosal n
F lacerum
Middle ear
Facial (VII) from stylo-mastoid F
Va
Vc
Lesser petrosal n
Petrotympanic fissure
Chorda tympani
Facial artery
Ophthalmic artery
Lacrimal artery
Sup III
Inf III
Sup orbital fissure
Naso-ciliary n
Tendinous ring
Vb
Lingual n
Auriculo-temporal n
Middle meningeal art
Otic ganglion
To submandibular gland
To sublingual gland
Levator palpebrae superioris
Long ciliary ns
Short ciliary ns
Ciliary ganglion hanging from n to inf oblique
N to medial pterygoid
Tensor palati
Tensor tympani
To parotid gland
Lacrimal n
Lacrimal gland
Foramen rotundum
Pterygopalatine fossa
Pharyngeal br of Vb
Naso-palatine n
Gtr & lssr palatine ns
Link from maxillary (Vb) to lacrimal (Va)
Zygomatico-temporal n
Zygomatico-facial n
Infra-orbital n
Middle/ant alveolar ns
Post sup alveolar n
Pterygomaxillary fissure

* **N of pterygoid canal**

Summary of taste

The sensation of taste originates in taste buds in the mucosa of the tongue and oropharynx. The buds are surrounded by the endings of the gustatory nerves which transmit taste as special visceral afferent sensation to the nucleus of the tractus solitarius in the brain stem. The three cranial nerves involved are facial (VII), glossopharyngeal (IX) and vagus (X) and the cell bodies for taste are in the geniculate, inferior glossopharyngeal and inferior vagal ganglia respectively.

Taste buds are found as follows:
1 As single buds in the mucosa.
2 In fungiform papillae on the anterior two-thirds of the tongue.
3 In the grooves around vallate papillae which are just anterior to the sulcus terminalis of the tongue.
4 In foliate papillae on the sides of the anterior two-thirds of the tongue.

4

Position of taste bud	Type of bud (1, 2, 3, 4 as above)	Nerve supply
Anterior two-thirds of tongue	1, 2, 4	Chorda tympani (VII) Carried by lingual N _also sublingual and_
Associated with posterior third of tongue	1, 3	Glossopharyngeal
Posterior wall of oropharynx	1	Glossopharyngeal
Palatoglossal arches	1	Glossopharyngeal
Oral aspect of soft palate	1	Lesser palatine (maxillary division of trigeminal) and glossopharyngeal
Anterior surface of epiglottis and valleculae	1	Internal laryngeal branch of superior laryngeal nerve (vagus)

Distribution of parasympathetics of head and neck

This complex for reference only diagram is for those who want to see the global arrangement of the parasympathetics in the neck and head. Parasympathetics are shown in red. Cranial nerves carrying the pre- or postganglionic fibres are shown in black. Sympathetics are shown in yellow. Interrupted yellow lines indicate probable additional pathways for sympathetics (see p. 82, left hand page)

ganglia :
geniculate ; inferior glossopharyngeal , inferior vagal
VII   IX   X

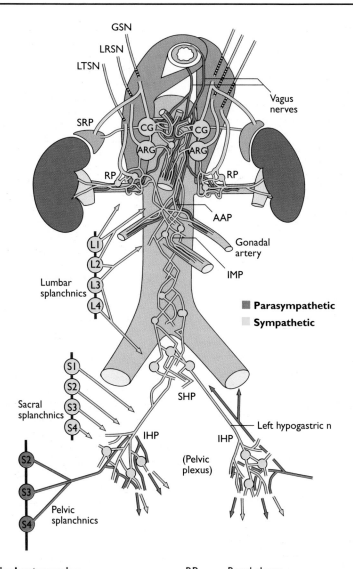

Abdominal autonomics

GSN	Greater splanchnic nerve
LRSN	Lesser splanchnic nerve
LTSN	Least splanchnic nerve
CG	Coeliac ganglion
ARG	Aorticorenal ganglion
RP	Renal plexus
SRP	Suprarenal plexus
AAP	Abdominal aortic plexus
IMP	Inferior mesenteric plexus
SHP	Superior hypogastric plexus
IHP	Inferior hypogastric plexus

Abdominal autonomics

The **greater splanchnic nerve** (T5–9) supplies the coeliac and aorticorenal ganglia and the suprarenal gland with preganglionic sympathetic fibres.

The **lesser splanchnic nerve** (T10,11) supplies the aorticorenal ganglion with similar fibres.

The **least splanchnic nerve** (T12) supplies the renal plexus with similar fibres.

Each of the splanchnic nerves pierces the crura of the diaphragm to enter the abdomen. They each carry efferent and afferent fibres.

The **coeliac ganglia** lie on each side of the coeliac trunk. They are supplied by preganglionic sympathetic fibres from the greater splanchnic nerves. Postganglionic sympathetic fibres leave these ganglia and form the coeliac plexus.

The **coeliac plexus** connects the coeliac ganglia across the midline; it surrounds the coeliac truck and extends down to become the superior mesenteric plexus. The coeliac plexus also receives preganglionic parasympathetic fibres from the vagus nerves. The fate of these fibres, both sympathetic and parasympathetic, is twofold. Many leave the plexus on branches of the coeliac trunk to be distributed to the bowel and other organs such as liver and spleen. Others pass downwards to reach other plexuses before being distributed similarly.

The **aorticorenal ganglia** are partially detached parts of the coeliac ganglia, lying just inferiorly. They contribute to both the coeliac and renal plexuses. As with the coeliac ganglia, sympathetic fibres leaving these ganglia are postganglionic.

A **renal plexus** surrounds the beginning of each renal artery. It has postganglionic sympathetic contributions from the coeliac and aorticorenal ganglia and preganglionic contributions from the least splanchnic nerve and the first lumbar splanchnic nerve. It has a few small ganglia for these preganglionic fibres to synapse. In addition it has both sympathetic and parasympathetic contributions from the coeliac and abdominal aortic plexuses. It supplies mainly the kidney and upper ureter with sympathetic and parasympathetic fibres although the function of the latter fibres is not clear.

The **superior mesenteric plexus** around the superior mesenteric artery is a downwards extension of the coeliac plexus. Its mixed sympathetic and parasympathetic fibres are distributed on this artery.

The **abdominal aortic (intermesenteric) plexus** lies on the aorta between the superior and inferior mesenteric arteries. It is connected above to the coeliac ganglia and plexus, aorticorenal ganglia and vagus nerves; below, it is in continuity with the inferior mesenteric and superior hypogastric plexuses. It also has preganglionic sympathetic input from the first and second lumbar splanchnic nerves.

The **vagus nerves** enter the abdomen via the oesophageal opening and distribute to abdominal organs and the bowel as far as two-thirds along the transverse colon via the coeliac and superior mesenteric plexuses. These preganglionic fibres synapse in small ganglia in the walls of the organs or bowel.

The **inferior mesenteric plexus** surrounds the beginning of the inferior mesenteric artery and is supplied by the abdominal aortic plexus with additional preganglionic sympathetic input from the second and third lumbar splanchnic nerves. Parasympathetic fibres from the sacral outflow (S2,3,4) ascend via the left inferior and superior hypogastric plexuses to be distributed with the sympathetic fibres on branches of the inferior mesenteric artery.

The **suprarenal plexus** on each side is supplied by the greater splanchnic nerve and a branch from the coeliac ganglion. The majority of sympathetic fibres reaching it are preganglionic to the medulla. There is no parasympathetic supply to the suprarenal gland.

The **lumbar splanchnics** are sympathetic preganglionic fibres that leave the sympathetic chain to supplement the thoracic splanchnics. L1 joins the renal plexus, L1, L2 the abdominal aortic plexus, L2,L3 the inferior mesenteric plexus and L3,L4 the superior hypogastric plexus.

4

The **superior hypogastric plexus** lies over and just below the bifurcation of the aorta. It is supplied by fibres continuing down from the abdominal aortic plexus (postganglionic) and the third and fourth lumbar splanchnic nerves (preganglionic). It contains a few small ganglia before forming **left and right hypogastric nerves** which pass down to the inferior hypogastric plexuses. It supplies the iliac vessels via the iliac plexuses and the ureter. It also has pelvic parasympathetics (S2,3,4) ascending through it on the way to the inferior mesenteric artery to supply bowel from the left side of the transverse colon downwards.

There is an **inferior hypogastric plexus** on each side wall of the pelvis. The two together make the pelvic plexus. They are supplied by pre- and postganglionic sympathetic fibres running in the hypogastric nerves from the superior hypogastric plexus and are supplemented by the first and second sacral splanchnics (preganglionic sympathetic) and the pelvic splanchnics (parasympathetic). They contain small ganglia for the synapses of any remaining preganglionic sympathetic fibres. The postganglionic sympathetic outflow from this plexus runs on arteries to give vasomotor supply and motor fibres to vas, seminal vesicles, prostate, anal and bladder sphincters and to inhibit peristalsis. Sympathetic sensory fibres arise in the upper rectum and body of uterus.

The **sacral splanchnics** are sympathetic preganglionic fibres that leave the sympathetic chain to supplement the pelvic sympathetics. S1 and S2 join the pelvic plexus or hypogastric nerve on each side. S3 and S4 from each side form a plexus on the median sacral artery.

The **pelvic splanchnics** are the caudal parasympathetic outflow (S2,3,4) and these fibres join the inferior hypogastric plexuses before distribution either on arteries or lying free in the retroperitoneum. The fibres are preganglionic and synapse in the walls of the organs they supply. They are motor to large bowel beyond the left third of the transverse colon, bladder and uterus. They are also sensory to some pelvic organs (bladder, proximal urethra, ampulla of rectum, anal canal, cervix of uterus, upper vagina and prostate). Ascending mostly from the left inferior hypogastric plexus, are those fibres mentioned above that supply parasympathetics to the left large bowel beyond the distribution of the vagus. Some of these fibres pass through the superior hypogastric plexus and then the inferior mesenteric plexus to reach the inferior mesenteric artery, whilst others may run directly to the left colon via the retroperitoneum.

Notes:
1 The neurotransmitter substance is acetylcholine at the endings of all preganglionic autonomic nerves whether sympathetic or parasympathetic and also at the postganglionic parasympathetic endings. All these endings are termed cholinergic. All postganglionic sympathetic endings have either noradrenalin or adrenalin as the neurotransmitter except sweat glands which are cholinergic.
2 Unless mentioned above as specific actions, the sympathetic efferent (motor) fibres cause vasoconstriction, inhibit intestinal peristalsis and glandular activity. The parasympathetic efferent (motor) fibres, however, cause glandular secretion and intestinal peristalsis but are inhibitory to the pyloric and ileocaecal sphincters. There are also specific actions of penile/clitoral erection and contraction of the bladder and uterus.

Note: Apart from cranial nerves I and II, which clearly arise from specific sensory areas and their fibres pass directly to the brain, a nomenclature has been used to describe each nerve as arising centrally in the brain and passing out to its terminal branches irrespective of whether the nerve carries sensory, motor or a combination of fibres. Sympathetics have generally been omitted except in association with cranial nerves III and Va where they have specific functions and are carried by a branch of the cranial nerve.

Colour coding in figures
- Somatic motor—black
- Somatic sensory—black
- Special visceral motor (branchial muscles) —blue
- Special visceral sensory (taste and arterial receptors)—green
- General visceral motor (parasympathetic)—red
- General visceral sensory (parasympathetic)—green
- Special senses—black
- Sympathetic—yellow

5

Summary table of nuclei & fibres of cranial nerves

	Somatic motor	Special visceral motor (branchial)	General visceral motor (parasympathetic)	General visceral sensory	Special visceral sensory	Somatic sensory	Special senses
I							Smell **Limbic system**
II							Sight **Lat geniculate body**
III	**Nu: Oculomotor** Recti (sup, med, inf), inf oblique, levator palpebrae superioris		**Nu: Edinger–Westphal** *Ciliary ganglion* Ciliary body & muscle, sphincter pupillae				
IV	**Nu: Trochlear** Sup oblique						
V		**Nu: Motor of trigeminal** M of mastication, mylohyoid, ant digastric, tensors palati & tympani				**Nu: Sensory of V** Mesencephalic: proprioception Main: touch Spinal: pain & temperature For V (face, orbit, tongue)	
VI	**Nu: Abducent** Lat rectus						
VII		**Nu: Facial** M of facial expression, buccinator, post digastric, stylohyoid, stapedius	**Nu: Sup salivary** *Pterygopalatine & submandibular ganglia* Lacrimal, submandibular, sublingual & palatine glands		**Nu: Solitarius** Chorda tympani Taste: ant 2/3 tongue	**Nu: Sensory of V** Some skin of ext auditory meatus & tympanic membrane	
VIII							Hearing: 2 Nu Equilib: 4 Nu
IX		**Nu: Ambiguus** Stylopharyngeus	**Nu: Inf salivary** *Otic ganglion* Parotid, glands in post 1/3 tongue & oropharynx		**Nu: Solitarius** Taste: post 1/3 tongue, vallate papillae, oropharynx; baro- & chemoreceptors	**Nu: Sensory of V** Post 1/3 tongue, palate, pharynx, tonsil, middle ear	
X		**Nu: Ambiguus** M of pharynx, upper oesophagus, palate, larynx (from cranial XI)	**Nu: Dorsal motor of vagus** Cardiac & visceral muscle in thorax & abdomen	**Nu: Solitarius or dorsal sensory of vagus** From heart, lungs & abdominal viscera	**Nu: Solitarius** Taste: vallecula & epiglottis; baro- & chemoreceptors	**Nu: Sensory of V** Small area of skin behind auricle, in ext auditory meatus & on ear drum; pharynx; larynx	
XI	**Nu: Lat roots C1–5** Sternocleidomastoid & trapezius	**Nu: Ambiguus** M of palate & pharynx via vagus					
XII	**Nu: Hypoglossal** M of tongue (not palatoglossus)						
NB	Motor nuclei for skeletal muscle Cell bodies in CNS	Motor to muscles of branchial origin. Cell bodies in CNS	Motor nerves synapse in parasympathetic ganglia	From heart, lungs & gut	Taste: baro- & chemoreceptors	From skin & membranes. Cell bodies outside CNS except mesencephalic nu.	

All sensory fibres relay to: motor nuclei, cerebellum, opposite thalamus → sensory cortex

CNS = central nervous system; M = muscles; Nu = nucleus

5

POSTERIOR

Int carotid
artery

Foramen
lacerum

IV

VI

V

III

Vc

II

Va

Vb

ovale

rotundum

Superior orbital fissure

Sup
ophthalmic vein

Inferior
orbital
fissure

Lacrimal

Frontal

IV
III

Nasociliary

VI
III

Inf
ophthalmic
vein

ANTERIOR

Lateral view of left cavernous sinus as a simplified box shape

Olfactory nerve (I)

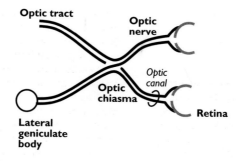

Optic nerve (II)

OLFACTORY NERVE (I)

From: Olfactory epithelium
To: Olfactory cortex
Contains: Special sense (smell)

The olfactory epithelium lines the superior surface of the superior concha, upper medial nasal septum and inferior surface of the cribriform plate of the ethmoid bone. The fibres of the olfactory cells run in the submucosa to pass through the cribriform plate of the ethmoid bone where they synapse in the olfactory bulb which lies on its superior surface. The bulb leads posteriorly to the olfactory tract which lies in the anterior cranial fossa on the inferior surface of the frontal lobe and conveys fibres to the anterior olfactory nucleus (in the posterior aspect of the olfactory bulb), to the prepiriform cortex, anterior perforating substance and septal areas.

OPTIC NERVE (II)

From: Retina
To: Lateral geniculate body
Contains: Special sense (sight)

The ganglion cells of the retina pass fibres out of the globe of the eye via the optic disc to enter the optic N which passes through the orbit within the dural sheath and within the cone of muscles. The nerve passes through the optic canal in the body of the sphenoid bone into the middle cranial fossa where it lies medial to the anterior clinoid process. The ophthalmic artery lies inferior to it in the canal and runs forwards to pierce the dura around the nerve inferomedially about 1 cm behind the eyeball. The nerve continues posteriorly at first lateral to, then superior to, the sella turcica where it forms the optic chiasma. Fibres from both eyes are distributed to each optic tract with medial retinal fibres (temporal visual fields) crossing to the opposite side. Each tract passes from the posterolateral angle of the chiasma, lying lateral to the pituitary infundibulum, to run lateral to the cerebral peduncle and medial to the uncus of the temporal lobe to reach the lateral geniculate body.

5

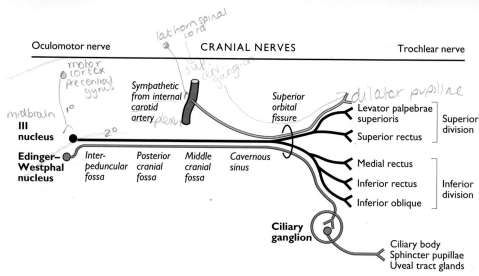

Handwritten annotations on diagram:
- lat horn spinal cord
- sup cerv ganglion
- motor cortex precentral gyrus
- midbrain 1°
- 2°
- plexus
- dilator pupillae

Oculomotor nerve (III)

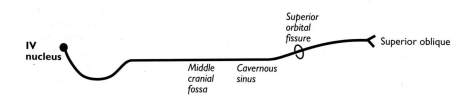

Trochlear nerve (IV)

Handwritten notes:

CN III IV VI LMN

- cavernous sinus → ant. med/lat wall
- emerge from C.S. → (S.O.f) → orbit
  ↓
  E.O. muscles.

OCULOMOTOR NERVE (III)
From: Oculomotor nucleus (somatic motor) and Edinger–Westphal nucleus (general visceral motor), ventral to cranial part of aqueduct in midbrain
To: Terminal brs
Contains: Somatic motor & general visceral motor

This nerve emerges medial to the cerebral peduncle in the interpeduncular fossa to reach the middle cranial fossa. It runs forward in close lateral relation to the posterior communicating artery below the margin of the tentorium cerebelli. It pierces the dura lateral to the posterior clinoid process to enter the roof of the cavernous sinus lying initially high in its lateral wall. It descends, passing medially over the trochlear N and

nasociliary branch of the ophthalmic division of the trigeminal N. It then enters the orbit through the superior orbital fissure within the tendinous ring having divided into superior and inferior divisions at the anterior end of the cavernous sinus. The superior division runs lateral to the optic N on the inferior surface of the superior rectus, passing through this muscle to terminate in levator palpebrae superioris. This division carries sympathetic supply to this muscle from the internal carotid artery in the cavernous sinus. The inferior division divides into terminal branches shortly after passing through the tendinous ring, the nerve to inferior oblique carrying the general visceral motor fibres (parasympathetic) to the ciliary ganglion. This lies posteriorly in the orbit inferolateral to the optic N.

TROCHLEAR NERVE (IV)
From: Trochlear nucleus in floor of aqueduct in dorsal midbrain, level with upper part of inferior colliculus
To: Terminal brs
Contains: Somatic motor

The fibres decussate within the substance of the midbrain to appear on the opposite side. The nerve emerges dorsally and passes lateral to the superior cerebellar peduncle then around the lateral aspect of the midbrain in the middle cranial fossa to lie

just above the superior border of the pons. It runs below the edge of the tentorium cerebelli between the posterior cerebral and the superior cerebellar arteries. It enters the roof of the cavernous sinus then onto its lateral wall where it is crossed medially by the oculomotor N from above down before entering the orbit through the superior orbital fissure superolateral to the tendinous ring. It runs medially above levator palpebrae superioris to terminate as it pierces superior oblique.

5

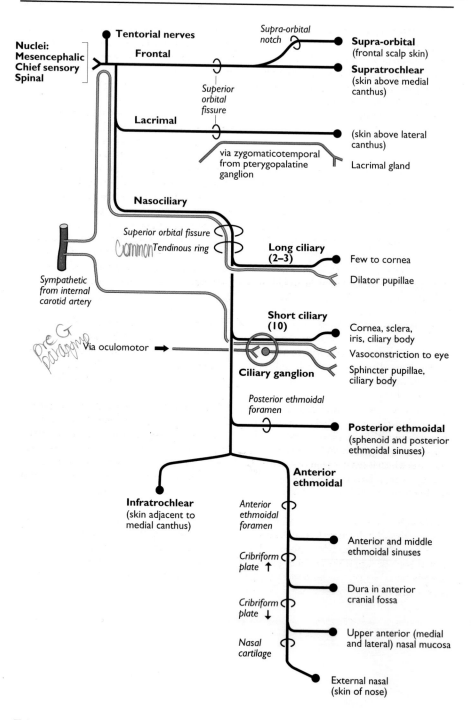

Trigeminal nerve—ophthalmic division (Va)

TRIGEMINAL NERVE—OPHTHALMIC DIVISION (Va)

From: Terminal nuclei are chief sensory (touch), mesencephalic (proprioception) and spinal (pain & temperature). They lie in pons, midbrain & medulla/upper cervical cord respectively

To: Terminal brs

Contains: Somatic sensory

The sensory root of the trigeminal N emerges from the ventral surface of the upper pons to enter the middle cranial fossa from where it passes to the trigeminal ganglion which lies in Meckel's cave, a prolongation of dura at the apex of the petrous temporal bone. The ophthalmic division leaves the trigeminal ganglion and runs forward in the lateral wall of the cavernous sinus below the trochlear N and is crossed medially by the oculomotor N. It divides into three terminal branches which pass through the superior orbital fissure separately. (Note: the mesencephalic nucleus is unusual in that it receives primary neurones that do not have the cell bodies in the ganglion but in the nucleus itself.)

Frontal N. Runs superolateral to the tendinous ring into the orbit where it continues forwards and medially above levator palpebrae superioris, to divide into terminal branches which leave the orbit over its superior margin through similarly named notches.

Lacrimal N. Runs lateral to the tendinous ring into the orbit. It passes laterally, close to the periosteum of the orbital plate of the frontal bone, to supply the lacrimal gland and adjoining conjunctiva. It then leaves the orbit over its superolateral margin to supply the lateral upper eyelid. In its course it carries parasympathetic fibres from the zygomatico-temporal branch of the maxillary N (Vb) to the lacrimal gland and sympathetic fibres from the nearby lacrimal artery.

Nasociliary N. Runs within the tendinous ring between superior and inferior division of the oculomotor N, crossing superior to the optic N to lie over the medial rectus. It leaves the muscular cone giving terminal branches before running through the anterior ethmoidal foramen in the ethmoid bone on the medial orbital wall as the anterior ethmoidal N. It traverses the anterior ethmoid sinus to run through its roof and onto the superior surface of the cribriform plate beneath the dura of the anterior cranial fossa. It passes through the plate again lateral to the crista galli onto the medial wall of the nose, first on the perpendicular plate of the ethmoid and then on the inner surface of the nasal bone. It passes into the skin of the nose beneath the inferior margin of the nasal bone as its terminal branch—the external nasal N.

Short ciliary Ns. Each of these 8–10 nerves emerges from the ciliary ganglion with a sensory component from the nasociliary N, postganglionic parasympathetic fibres from the oculomotor N and sympathetic fibres which pass directly from the internal carotid artery in the cavernous sinus.

Long ciliary Ns. Each of the 2–3 nerves has sensory fibres from the nasociliary N and sympathetic fibres for the dilator pupillae that are carried by the nasociliary N from the internal carotid artery in the cavernous sinus.

5

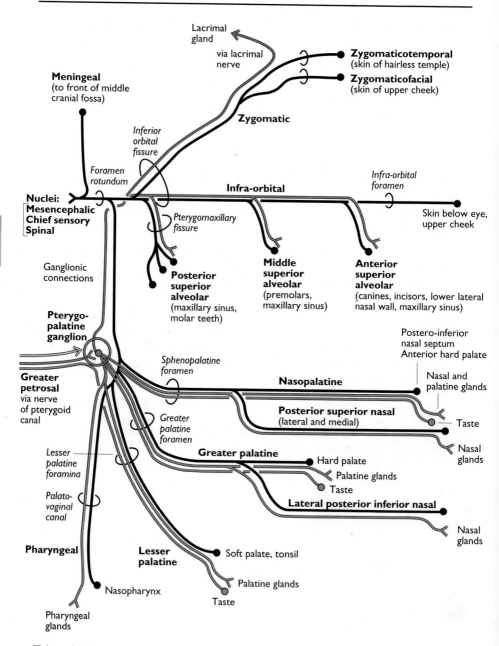

Lacrimal
gland

via lacrimal
nerve

Zygomaticotemporal
(skin of hairless temple)

Zygomaticofacial
(skin of upper cheek)

Meningeal
(to front of middle
cranial fossa)

*Inferior
orbital
fissure*

Zygomatic

*Foramen
rotundum*

Infra-orbital

*Infra-orbital
foramen*

Nuclei:
Mesencephalic
Chief sensory
Spinal

*Pterygomaxillary
fissure*

Skin below eye,
upper cheek

Ganglionic
connections

**Posterior
superior
alveolar**
(maxillary sinus,
molar teeth)

**Middle
superior
alveolar**
(premolars,
maxillary sinus)

**Anterior
superior
alveolar**
(canines, incisors, lower lateral
nasal wall, maxillary sinus)

**Pterygo-
palatine
ganglion**

*Sphenopalatine
foramen*

Postero-inferior
nasal septum
Anterior hard palate

**Greater
petrosal**
via nerve
of pterygoid
canal

Nasopalatine

Nasal and
palatine glands

Posterior superior nasal
(lateral and medial)

Taste

*Greater
palatine
foramen*

Nasal
glands

*Lesser
palatine
foramina*

Greater palatine

Hard palate

Palatine glands

Taste

*Palato-
vaginal
canal*

Lateral posterior inferior nasal

Nasal
glands

Pharyngeal

**Lesser
palatine**

Soft palate, tonsil

Nasopharynx

Palatine glands

Taste

Pharyngeal
glands

Trigeminal nerve—maxillary division (Vb)

TRIGEMINAL NERVE—MAXILLARY DIVISION (Vb)

From: Terminal nuclei are chief sensory (touch), mesencephalic (proprioception) and spinal (pain & temperature). They lie in pons, midbrain & medulla/upper cervical cord respectively

To: Terminal brs

Contains: Somatic sensory

(See ophthalmic division for course to the trigeminal ganglion.) The nerve leaves the ganglion to run low down in the lateral wall of the cavernous sinus before passing onto the floor of the middle cranial fossa and it then exits through the foramen rotundum in the greater wing of the sphenoid bone. It runs into the upper pterygopalatine fossa, giving branches via the pterygopalatine ganglion before passing into the orbit via the inferior orbital fissure to become the infra-orbital N. The pterygopalatine ganglion is suspended from the maxillary N by one or two roots and receives parasympathetic fibres from the greater petrosal N in the pterygopalatine fossa which are distributed with the terminal branches as shown.

Infra-orbital N. Passes laterally across the posterior aspect of the palatine bone and maxilla to pass through the inferior orbital fissure and to run into the infra-orbital groove in the orbital surface of the maxilla. It terminates in branches in the skin of the face having passed through the infra-orbital foramen which is the completed continuation of the infra-orbital groove.

Zygomatic N. Passes superiorly out of the pterygopalatine fossa through the inferior orbital fissure to run in the lateral orbit outside the cone of muscles. It terminates on the lateral orbital wall as facial and temporal branches which pass through unnamed canals in the zygomatic bone to reach the skin over the zygomatic bone and hairless temple respectively.

Nasopalatine (previously sphenopalatine) N. Passes through the sphenopalatine foramen to enter the posterior upper nasal cavity to end as terminal branches.

Pharyngeal N. A few fine branches of this nerve pass from the pterygopalatine ganglion into the orbit via the inferior orbital fissure to supply sensation and secretomotor fibres to the sphenoidal and ethmoidal sinuses.

Note: Other branches pass through foramina as indicated. Sympathetics have been omitted from the distribution of the pterygopalatine ganglion to avoid complicating the diagram.

5

Trigeminal nerve—mandibular division (Vc)

TRIGEMINAL NERVE—MANDIBULAR DIVISION (Vc)

From: Terminal nuclei are chief sensory (touch), mesencephalic (proprioception) and spinal (pain & temperature). They lie in pons, midbrain & medulla/upper cervical cord respectively. Motor nucleus (branchial muscles) is in upper pons

To: Terminal brs

Contains: Somatic sensory & special visceral motor

(See ophthalmic division for course to the trigeminal ganglion.) The smaller motor root leaves the ventral pons anteromedial to the sensory root. The sensory root leaves the ganglion from its lateral part and passes, after a short course over the greater wing of the sphenoid bone, through the foramen ovale. The motor root passes under the ganglion and unites with the sensory root just beyond the foramen ovale. The nerve that is so formed passes into the infratemporal fossa between tensor veli palatini and lateral pterygoid. It has a short course of 3–4mm before dividing into anterior and posterior divisions which provide terminal branches.

Anterior division

Deep temporal Ns. Usually two, run above the lateral pterygoid, over the infratemporal crest and on the squamous temporal and greater wing of the sphenoid bones deep to temporalis to supply it. They lie with their associated vessels deeply in the temporal fossa.

Lateral pterygoid Ns. Pierce the muscle directly to supply it.

Masseter N. Runs laterally over the lateral pterygoid and over the mandibular notch to pierce the deep surface of the muscle to supply it and the temporomandibular joint.

Buccal N. Runs forward over lateral pterygoid and lies deep to temporalis, the mandible and masseter. It runs through buccinator to supply a small area of overlying skin. The nerve is sensory only.

Posterior division

Auriculotemporal N. Passes posteriorly, briefly dividing to encircle the middle meningeal artery, before running between the neck of the mandible and the spheno-mandibular ligament. It winds around the neck of the mandible to pass laterally then superiorly lying between the temporo-mandibular joint and the external auditory meatus deep to the parotid gland. It terminates at the upper border of the gland as branches. The nerve receives general visceral motor fibres (parasympathetic) from the lesser petrosal N via the otic ganglion which lies suspended from the nerve to tensor tympani near the foramen ovale.

Lingual N. Passes forward and inferiorly to lie between lateral pterygoid and tensor veli palatini, then between medial pterygoid and the ramus of the mandible. It lies just beneath the mucous membrane of the mouth posteromedial to the third molar tooth. It passes lateral to styloglossus and hyoglossus and runs at first lateral, then inferior and then medial to the submandibular duct. It terminates over the lateral aspect of the anterior two-thirds of the tongue. It is joined 2cm anterior and inferior to the foramen ovale by general visceral motor and special visceral sensory fibres of the chorda tympani which relay in the submandibular ganglion. This ganglion which is suspended from the nerve by two roots lies on hyoglossus above the submandibular gland.

Inferior alveolar N. Passes deep to lateral pterygoid to lie between the spheno-mandibular ligament and the ramus of the mandible before entering the mandible via the inferior alveolar foramen. It terminates as cutaneous branches reappearing through the mental foramen in the anterior body of the mandible. The N to mylohyoid arises just before it enters the inferior alveolar foramen and pierces the sphenomandibular ligament to run in a groove on the medial surface of the body of the mandible below mylohyoid.

5

Abducent nerve (VI)

ABDUCENT NERVE (VI)

From: Abducent nucleus in sup part of floor
  of 4th ventricle in lower pons
To: Terminal brs
Contains: Somatic motor

The fibres leave the pons at its lower border above the pyramid of the medulla. It traverses the pontine basal cistern running forwards and superiorly to pierce the dura over the clivus inferolateral to the dorsum sellae. It arches forward directly over the ridge of the petrous temporal bone passing through the medial wall of the inferior petrosal sinus under the petroclinoid ligament and runs into the cavernous sinus. Here it lies directly lateral to the internal carotid artery before passing into the orbit through the superior orbital fissure within the tendinous ring. It passes forward and laterally to sink into the medial surface of the lateral rectus muscle.

5

Superior salivary nucleus

Nucleus solitarius

Sensory nucleus of V

Motor nucleus of VII

Nervus intermedius

Internal auditory meatus

Deep petrosal nerve
(sympathetic from internal carotid)

Greater petrosal

Petrous bone

Foramen lacerum

Middle cranial fossa

Pterygoid canal

Pterygopalatine ganglion

Glands:
Lacrimal
Nasal
Palatine
Pharyngeal

Palatine taste buds

Geniculate ganglion

External auditory meatus

Stapedius

Petro-tympanic fissure

Chorda tympani

Submandibular ganglion

Submandibular Sublingual glands

Taste: anterior 2/3 tongue

Stylomastoid foramen

Posterior auricular

Occipito-frontalis
Auricularis

Posterior belly of digastric
Stylohyoid

Parotid gland

Temporal   Corrugator
Orbicularis oculi
Occipitofrontalis

Zygomatic 1
Zygomatic 2   Orbicularis oculi

Buccal   Levator labii superioris
Levator anguli oris
Buccinator
Orbicularis oris
Zygomaticus major & minor
Nasalis
Procerus
Levator labii superioris
   alaeque nasi

Mandibular   Mentalis
Depressor anguli oris
Depressor labii inferioris
Risorius

Cervical   Platysma

Facial nerve (VII)

Temporal	Two
Zygomatic	Zulus
Buccal	Buggered
Mandibular	my
Cervical	cat.

FACIAL NERVE (VII)

From: Facial motor nucleus deep to reticular formation in lower pons. Sup salivary nucleus (general visceral motor) distal to motor nucleus. Gustatory nucleus (taste) in superior end of nucleus solitarius in medulla. Sensory nucleus of V (see trigeminal N)

To: Terminal brs

Contains: Somatic sensory, special visceral sensory & motor, general visceral motor

It leaves the pons at the cerebellopontine angle medial to the vestibulocochlear N (VIII) as two nerve roots—the facial motor root and the nervus intermedius. The nervus intermedius contains special visceral sensory, general visceral motor and somatic sensory fibres which connect with gustatory, superior salivary and sensory trigeminal nuclei respectively. These two roots pass across the subarachnoid space together to enter the internal auditory meatus and pass laterally along it to reach and enter the facial canal. The two roots then unite and pass laterally onto the medial wall of the middle ear before turning 90 degrees posteriorly at the geniculate ganglion. It continues posteriorly running above the promontory and oval window and below the lateral semicircular canal. Finally the nerve turns 90 degrees inferiorly to run down in the medial wall of the aditus of the mastoid antrum. It leaves the middle ear via the stylomastoid foramen to pass between the mastoid process and the tympanic ring before passing between the deep and superficial portions of the parotid gland. Within the gland it lies superficial to the styloid process, retromandibular vein and external carotid artery before dividing into terminal branches which leave just medial to the anterior border of the gland.

Greater petrosal N. Arises from the main nerve at the geniculate ganglion and passes medially through the petrous temporal bone to lie in a groove on its anterior surface beneath the temporal lobe and dura of the middle cranial fossa. It runs beneath the trigeminal ganglion and then passes anteromedially but lying anterolateral to the internal carotid artery as this vessel emerges across the upper end of foramen lacerum. It is joined by the deep petrosal N (sympathetic) off the artery and this combined nerve (the N of the pterygoid canal or Vidian's N) passes into the same named canal which commences a short way into the anterior wall of the foramen lacerum at the root of the pterygoid process of the sphenoid. This canal exits into the pterygopalatine fossa where the nerve enters the posterior aspect of the pterygopalatine ganglion and distributes its fibres with branches of the maxillary division (Vb) of the trigeminal N.

Chorda tympani. Arises from the facial nerve in the facial canal during its descent from the medial wall of the middle ear. It runs back into the middle ear on the posterior wall before passing anteriorly between the two layers of the flaccid part of the tympanic membrane and over the handle of the malleus. It leaves the middle ear by passing into the petrous temporal bone and emerges via the petrotympanic fissure to pass into the infratemporal fossa medial to the spine of the sphenoid bone which it grooves. It runs antero-inferiorly, deep to lateral pterygoid, to join the lingual branch of the mandibular division (Vc) 2 cm below the skull.

Nuclei:
Cochlear — Cochlea

Vestibular — Semicircular canals & utricle
Saccule

Vestibulocochlear nerve (VIII)

Inferior salivary nucleus

Sensory nucleus of V

Nucleus ambiguus

Nucleus solitarius

Inferior ganglion of IX

Dura of posterior cranial fossa

Anterior compartment of jugular foramen

Tympanic branch

Middle ear

Lesser petrosal

Petrous bone

Otic ganglion

Foramen ovale

Parotid gland

Petrous bone

Middle ear

Sympathetic off middle meningeal artery

Stylopharyngeus

Tonsil

→ plexus (sen.)

Pharyngeal (mucosa of oropharynx)

Lingual ⎤ Posterior
Taste ⎦ 1/3 tongue

Carotid (carotid sinus and body)

Glossopharyngeal nerve (IX)

VESTIBULOCOCHLEAR NERVE (VIII)

From: 4 Vestibular & 2 cochlear nuclei in floor of 4th ventricle in pons
To: Inner ear
Contains: Special sense (hearing, balance)

It emerges at the cerebellopontine angle as a single nerve and traverses the subarachnoid space to enter the internal auditory meatus where the cochlear element separates and pierces the temporal bone in its antero-inferior quadrant. The vestibular element divides into upper and lower divisions to pierce the temporal bone in its postero-superior and postero-inferior quadrants. The cochlear N runs in the cochlear modiolus to end in terminal connections. The upper vestibular division runs to supply the semi-circular canals and the utricle, the lower division the saccule.

GLOSSOPHARYNGEAL NERVE (IX)

From: Sensory nucleus of V (common sensation—see trigeminal N). Nucleus solitarius (taste—medulla). Nucleus ambiguus (motor to branchial muscle—medulla). Inf salivary nucleus (secretomotor—lower pons)
To: Terminal brs
Contains: Somatic sensory, general & special visceral motor, special visceral sensory

The fibres leave the medulla as three or four rootlets lying posterior to the olive. They rapidly fuse into one nerve which passes anterolaterally into the anterior compartment of the jugular foramen (between petrous temporal and occipital bones). It passes lateral to the inferior petrosal sinus which separates it from the vagus and accessory Ns and runs anteriorly out of the compartment. It forms the glossopharyngeal ganglia below the compartment as it passes between internal jugular vein and internal carotid artery. It passes inferolaterally looping around the upper border of stylopharyngeus, runs deep to hyoglossus and terminates in lingual and pharyngeal branches.

Carotid N. Arises just below the ganglia and runs down closely adherent to the internal carotid artery within the carotid sheath to reach the carotid sinus and carotid body.

Lesser petrosal N. The tympanic branch (Jacobson's N) of the glossopharyngeal N arises just below the ganglia to pass via the petrous temporal bone into the middle ear. It mingles with parasympathetic fibres of the facial N (VII) and sympathetics from the internal carotid artery over the promontory on the medial wall to form the lesser petrosal N. This nerve then leaves the middle ear via the medial side of the roof and passes through the petrous temporal bone into the middle cranial fossa. Here it lies beneath the dura to run forward before passing through the foramen ovale and synapsing below in the otic ganglion in the infratemporal fossa. From here it is distributed with the auriculo-temporal branch of the mandibular division (Vc) to the parotid gland.

5

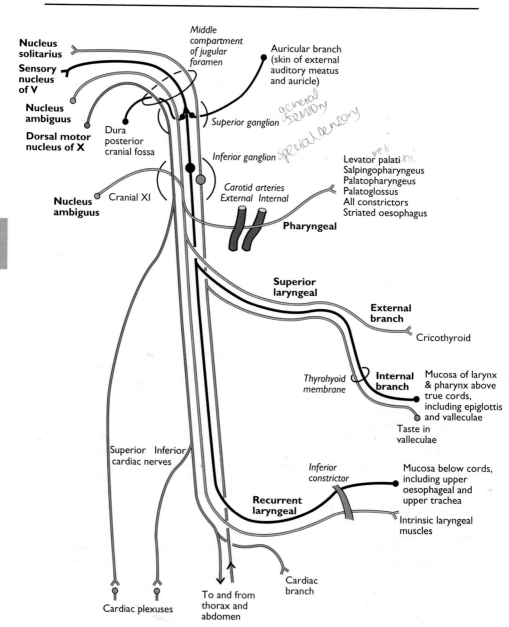

Middle
compartment
of jugular
foramen

**Nucleus
solitarius**

**Sensory
nucleus
of V**

**Nucleus
ambiguus**

**Dorsal motor
nucleus of X**

Dura
posterior
cranial fossa

Auricular branch
(skin of external
auditory meatus
and auricle)

Superior ganglion   general sensory

special sensory

Inferior ganglion

**Nucleus
ambiguus**   Cranial XI

*Carotid arteries
External Internal*

Levator palati
Salpingopharyngeus
Palatopharyngeus
Palatoglossus
All constrictors
Striated oesophagus

Pharyngeal

**Superior
laryngeal**

**External
branch**

Cricothyroid

*Thyrohyoid
membrane*

**Internal
branch**

Mucosa of larynx
& pharynx above
true cords,
including epiglottis
and valleculae

Taste in
valleculae

Superior   Inferior
cardiac nerves

*Inferior
constrictor*

Mucosa below cords,
including upper
oesophageal and
upper trachea

**Recurrent
laryngeal**

Intrinsic laryngeal
muscles

Cardiac
branch

Cardiac plexuses

To and from
thorax and
abdomen

Vagus nerve (X)

VAGUS NERVE (X)

From: Dorsal motor nucleus of vagus
(general visceral motor—lower medulla).
Nucleus ambiguus (branchial motor—
medulla). Nucleus solitarius (taste &
general visceral sensory—medulla).
Sensory nucleus of V (common sensation—
see trigeminal N)
To: Terminal brs
Contains: Somatic sensory, general & special
visceral sensory, general & special visceral
motor

The fibres emerge from the medulla as a
series of rootlets posterior to the olive
between the glossopharyngeal and cranial
accessory rootlets. These form into a single
nerve that passes into the middle compartment of the jugular foramen. Below the
foramen it forms superior and inferior
ganglia before being joined by the cranial
part of the accessory N. It passes vertically
down within the carotid sheath closely
related to the internal carotid artery and
lying between it and the internal jugular
vein.

Pharyngeal branch. Passes from the vagus
at the inferior ganglion running between
internal and external carotid arteries to
reach the lateral wall of the pharynx. These
fibres are mostly from the cranial part of the
accessory N.

Superior laryngeal N. Passes from the
inferior ganglion running steeply down
anteriorly, lying posterior and then medial
to the internal carotid artery. It pierces the
carotid sheath to run on the wall of the
pharynx to the level of the greater cornu of
the hyoid bone where it divides.

Internal branch. Runs down anteriorly onto
the thyrohyoid membrane which it pierces
at the level of the vallecula, and is then
distributed as terminal branches to the

mucous membrane of the vallecula and
larynx down to the vocal folds.

External branch. Runs down over the
inferior constrictor accompanied by the
superior thyroid artery to reach the
cricothyroid muscle.

Recurrent laryngeal N. In the neck the two
sides follow the same course ascending in
the tracheo-oesophageal groove. As the
nerve passes medial to the lateral lobe of the
thyroid gland it is intimately related to the
inferior thyroid artery. It passes beneath the
inferior border of cricopharyngeus (inferior
constrictor) to terminate within the submucosa of the larynx. The nerve on the right
originates from the vagus anterior to the
subclavian artery around which it hooks
posteriorly before running medially to
ascend in the tracheo-oesophageal groove.
The nerve on the left originates from the
vagus inferolateral to the arch of the aorta
passing inferior to the arch and posterior to
the ligamentum arteriosum. It runs to the
right of the arch as it passes posteriorly over
the left side of the trachea to reach the
tracheo-oesophageal groove.

Cardiac Ns. The upper branch arises below
the inferior ganglion and the lower branch
arises in the root of the neck. On the right
they pass down anterior to the brachiocephalic artery and on the left over the aortic
arch to terminate in the cardiac plexuses.

Note: General visceral motor (parasympathetic) and general visceral sensory
fibres in the vagus to and from the thorax
and abdomen arise/end in the dorsal motor
nucleus of vagus and nucleus solitarius
respectively.
  All branchial motor (special visceral
motor) fibres in the vagus which supply
muscles arise in the nucleus ambiguus but
the majority, if not all, are supplied to the
vagus by the cranial accessory (XI).

Accessory nerve (XI)

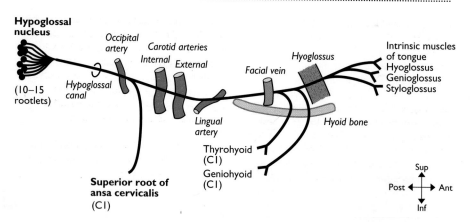

Hypoglossal nerve (XII)

ACCESSORY NERVE (XI)

From: Cranial root from nucleus ambiguus
(branchial motor—medulla). Spinal root
from spinal nuclei (C1–C5)

To: Terminal brs

Contains: Somatic motor (spinal), special
visceral motor (cranial)

The fibres of the cranial root emerge from
the medulla as four to six rootlets posterior
to the olive immediately below those of the
vagus to fuse into a single nerve. They are
joined by the spinal root as it ascends via
the foramen magnum (see cervical plexus,
pp. 112–113). The nerve passes out of the
posterior cranial fossa through the middle
compartment of the jugular foramen

posterior to the vagus and anterior to the
internal jugular vein. Inferior to the foramen
the cranial element passes inferomedially
to fuse with the vagus to which it adds its
complement of special visceral motor fibres.

Spinal root. Passes posterolaterally, usually
posterior to the internal jugular vein, over
the lateral mass of the atlas (C1) and deep to
the occipital artery to enter the deep surface
of sternocleidomastoid. It traverses the
posterior triangle of the neck from one-third
of the way down the posterior border of
sternocleidomastoid to one-third of the way
up the anterior border of trapezius where it
terminates.

HYPOGLOSSAL NERVE (XII)

From: Hypoglossal nucleus in floor of 4th
ventricle in medulla

To: Terminal brs

Contains: Somatic motor

Its fibres pass out of the anterolateral surface of the medulla between the olive and
pyramid as a series of 10–15 rootlets. These
fuse to form two roots which pass posterior
to the vertebral artery as they run into the
hypoglossal canal where they themselves

fuse. The nerve runs out of the canal anteriorly, lateral to the occipital, internal carotid,
external carotid and lingual arteries before
passing over the apex of the greater cornu
of the hyoid bone. It then runs anteriorly,
looping lateral to hyoglossus, deep to
mylohyoid, to end in terminal branches
beneath the submandibular gland.

Note: C1 fibres join the hypoglossal N (pp.
112–113). This is not shown in this diagram
but they are seen leaving it.

6: PERIPHERAL NERVES

6

POSTERIOR PRIMARY RAMI   *LATERAL ROOTS*   *ANTERIOR PRIMARY RAMI*

Spinal accessory

Sub-occipital

Hypoglossal (XII)

Rectus capitis posterior - major + minor

Obliquus capitis superior + inferior

Semispinalis capitis

Greater occipital (skin of posterior occiput)

Obliquus capitis inferior
Semispinalis capitis
Splenius
Longissimus capitis

C1

Superior root

Ansa cervicalis

C2

Inferior root

C3

C4

C5

Geniohyoid

Thyrohyoid

Omohyoid

Sternohyoid

Sternothyroid

Lesser occipital (skin of lower lateral occiput)

Great auricular (skin of lower auricle and angle of jaw)

Transverse cervical (skin of anterior neck)

Supraclavicular (skin of anterior lower neck, upper chest and shoulder)

Suprasternal

Supraclavicular

Supra-acromial

Phrenic

Cervical plexus (C1,2,3,4,5)

6

CERVICAL PLEXUS (C1,2,3,4,5)
From: C1,2,3,4,5 Ns
To: Ns as shown

It arises mostly from the anterior primary rami deep between scalenus medius and scalenus anterior at the level of C1–C4 vertebrae and is covered by prevertebral fascia lying deep to sternocleidomastoid. The cutaneous branches pierce the prevertebral fascia and run into the posterior triangle of the neck where they pierce the investing layer of the deep cervical fascia to terminate in subcutaneous Ns.

Ansa cervicalis (C1–C3). Superior root (anterior primary rami C1)—passes directly to the hypoglossal N (XII) between rectus capitis anterior and lateralis. It leaves the hypoglossal N lateral to the occipital artery and runs anterior to the internal and common carotid arteries where it joins the inferior root. Inferior root (anterior primary rami C2,3)—passes laterally around the internal jugular vein having pierced the prevertebral fascia at the level of C2/3. It runs forwards and anteriorly as a long loop to meet with the superior root anterior to the common carotid artery.

Suboccipital N (posterior primary ramus of C1). Emerges through the dura to run beneath the vertebral artery closely applied to the posterior arch of the atlas (C1). It pierces the posterior atlanto-occipital membrane between obliquus capitis superior and rectus capitis posterior major to terminate in muscular branches in the suboccipital triangle.

Greater occipital N (posterior primary rami of C2, and a small contribution from C3). Emerges from the posterior spinal dura at the intervertebral foramen and passes posteriorly over the transverse process of the axis (C2) below obliquus capitis inferior. It then winds around this muscle to ascend deep to semispinalis piercing it and trapezius near to their insertions into the superior nuchal line. It terminates as cutaneous branches running in the scalp with the occipital artery.

Spinal accessory N (XIs) (lateral roots C1–C5) is formed from the unique lateral roots of C1–C5 and ascends within the subarachnoid space lateral to the cord and posterior to the denticulate ligament, to pass through the foramen magnum posterior to the vertebral artery to meet with the cranial root.

Phrenic N (see pp. 124–125).

Great auricular N (C2,3). Supplies skin over parotid gland and angle of jaw (this is the only area of the face that is not supplied by a cranial nerve), lower lateral auricle below external auditory meatus, and whole of posterior (medial) auricle.

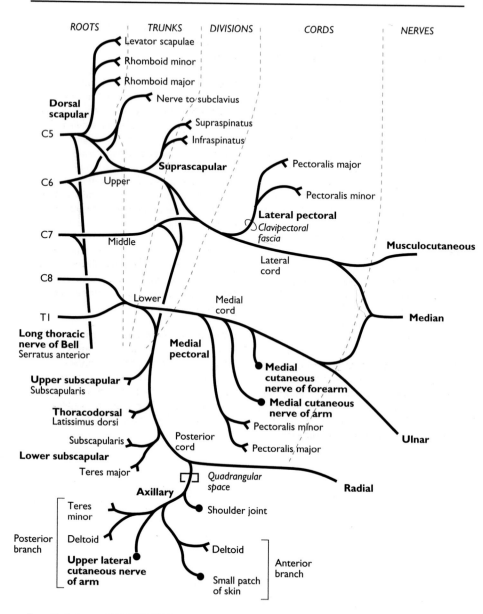

Brachial plexus (C5,6,7,8,T1)

BRACHIAL PLEXUS (C5,6,7,8,T1)
From: Ant primary rami of C5,6,7,8,T1
To: Musculocutaneous, median, ulnar &
    radial Ns

It emerges as five roots lying anterior to
scalenus medius and posterior to scalenus
anterior. The trunks lie in the base of the
posterior triangle of the neck, where they are
palpable, and pass over the 1st rib posterior
to the third part of subclavian artery to
descend to lie behind the clavicle. The
divisions form behind the middle third of the
clavicle lying on the upper fibres of serratus
anterior and around the axillary artery, as
they form the cords. The cords lie in the
axilla related to the second part of the
axillary artery lying medial, lateral and
posterior as their names indicate and
posterior to pectoralis minor. Terminal
nerves are formed around the third part of
the axillary artery posterior to the lower
fibres of pectoralis major.

Axillary N (C5,6). Arises posterior to the
third part of axillary artery. It runs
posteriorly on subscapularis to pass through
the quadrangular space with the posterior
circumflex humeral artery. It is intimately
related to the medial aspect of the surgical
neck of the humerus running laterally to end
in anterior and posterior divisions deep to
deltoid.

Upper lateral cutaneous N of arm. Is a
continuation of the posterior branch of the
axillary N and supplies skin over the lower
lateral deltoid. Damage to the axillary N
(and hence this nerve) gives a 'regimental
badge' area of sensory loss.

Thoracodorsal N (C5,6,7). Runs with the
subscapular artery down the medial scapular
border over teres major and into latissimus
dorsi.

Long thoracic N of Bell (C5,6,7). Descends
posterior to the trunks of the plexus and the
first part of the axillary artery to lie on the
lateral aspect of serratus anterior on the
medial axillary wall.

Suprascapular N (C5,6). Arises in the
posterior triangle of the neck, passes
posterolaterally deep to trapezius and
omohyoid and runs through the suprascapular notch into the supraspinous fossa.
It descends laterally around the scapular
spine into the infraspinous fossa.

6

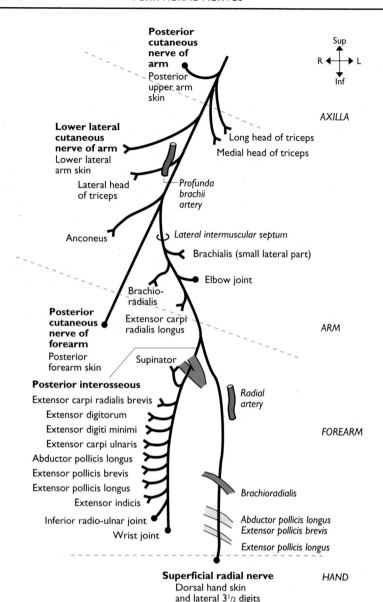

Posterior cutaneous nerve of arm
Posterior upper arm skin

AXILLA

Lower lateral cutaneous nerve of arm
Lower lateral arm skin

Long head of triceps
Medial head of triceps

Lateral head of triceps

Profunda brachii artery

Anconeus

Lateral intermuscular septum

Brachialis (small lateral part)

Elbow joint

Brachio-radialis

Extensor carpi radialis longus

ARM

Posterior cutaneous nerve of forearm
Posterior forearm skin

Supinator

Posterior interosseous
Extensor carpi radialis brevis
Extensor digitorum
Extensor digiti minimi
Extensor carpi ulnaris
Abductor pollicis longus
Extensor pollicis brevis
Extensor pollicis longus
Extensor indicis
Inferior radio-ulnar joint
Wrist joint

Radial artery

FOREARM

Brachioradialis

Abductor pollicis longus
Extensor pollicis brevis

Extensor pollicis longus

Superficial radial nerve
Dorsal hand skin
and lateral 3$^{1}/_{2}$ digits
short of the nail beds

HAND

Radial nerve (C5,6,7,8,T1)

6

RADIAL NERVE (C5,6,7,8,T1)
From: Post cord of brachial plexus
To: Terminal brs

It arises as the continuation of the posterior cord and descends posterior to the axillary and brachial arteries passing inferior to the tendons of latissimus dorsi and teres major to run with the profunda brachii artery between the long and medial heads of triceps and through the lateral triangular space. It gives off the posterior cutaneous N of arm before leaving the axilla. It then runs over the spiral line of the humerus between medial and lateral heads of triceps giving muscular and cutaneous branches, and pierces the lateral intermuscular septum at the mid point of the humerus to reach the anterior compartment. Here it lies deep to the upper fibres of brachialis then brachioradialis, before entering the lateral cubital fossa. It divides into terminal branches over the lateral epicondyle.

Superficial terminal branch. Runs over supinator, pronator teres and flexor digitorum superficialis and lies under brachioradialis running with the radial artery on its medial aspect from one-third of the way down the forearm. It passes posteriorly, emerging from under the tendon of brachioradialis proximal to the radial styloid and then passes over the tendons of the snuff box where it terminates as cutaneous branches to the dorsum of the hand.

Posterior interosseous N. Passes between the two heads of supinator three fingers' breadth below radial head passing into the posterior compartment where it breaks up into terminal muscular branches in the plane between the deep and superficial muscles in this compartment.

6

Sup

R ←→ L

Inf

Shoulder joint

Coracobrachialis

Coracobrachialis

Long head
of biceps

Short head
of biceps

Brachialis

Elbow joint

Biceps

ARM

FOREARM

Deep fascia

**Lateral cutaneous
nerve of forearm**
Lateral forearm skin

Musculocutaneous nerve (C5,6,7)

MUSCULOCUTANEOUS NERVE (C5,6,7)
From: Lat cord
To: Terminal brs

It arises obliquely behind the lower fibres of pectoralis minor lying lateral to the axillary artery and passes laterally between the two conjoined heads of coracobrachialis. It runs laterally downwards between biceps and brachialis, usually adherent to the deep surface of biceps. The terminal branch is the lateral cutaneous N of forearm.

Lateral cutaneous N of forearm. Emerges lateral to the tendon of biceps in the cubital fossa, piercing the deep fascia just below the elbow and descends over the lateral aspect of the forearm to terminate in the skin over the radial artery at the wrist.

6

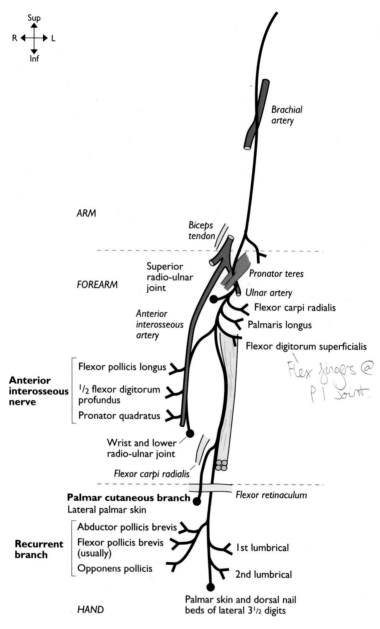

Sup
R ←――→ L
Inf

6

Brachial
artery

ARM

Biceps
tendon

Superior
radio-ulnar
joint

FOREARM

Anterior
interosseous
artery

Pronator teres

Ulnar artery

Flexor carpi radialis

Palmaris longus

Flexor digitorum superficialis

Flex fingers @
P I Joint.

**Anterior
interosseous
nerve**

Flexor pollicis longus

1/2 flexor digitorum
profundus

Pronator quadratus

Wrist and lower
radio-ulnar joint

Flexor carpi radialis

Palmar cutaneous branch
Lateral palmar skin

Flexor retinaculum

Abductor pollicis brevis

**Recurrent
branch**

Flexor pollicis brevis
(usually)

Opponens pollicis

1st lumbrical

2nd lumbrical

Palmar skin and dorsal nail
beds of lateral 3 1/2 digits

HAND

Median nerve (C6,7,8,T1)

MEDIAN NERVE (C6,7,8,T1)
From: Med & lat cords
To: Terminal brs

It is formed in the lower axilla by two roots (heads) which clasp the axillary artery. The nerve initially lies anterior to the axillary artery and then lateral to it and subsequently lateral to the brachial artery. The median N then crosses the brachial artery, usually anteriorly, at the level of the mid humerus, to lie medial to the artery in the cubital fossa. It lies first on coracobrachialis and then brachialis. It passes beneath the bicipital aponeurosis at the elbow leaving the cubital fossa between the two heads of pronator teres before crossing superficial to the ulnar artery and giving its anterior interosseous branch below this. It lies applied to the deep surface of flexor digitorum superficialis on flexor digitorum profundus. It emerges from the lateral side of flexor digitorum superficialis about 5 cm proximal to the wrist where it gives its palmar cutaneous branch and then passes deep to the flexor retinaculum between the tendons of flexor digitorum superficialis and flexor carpi radialis. In the carpal tunnel it divides into terminal branches—recurrent (muscular) branch and palmar digital Ns.

Anterior interosseous N. Arises just below the two heads of pronator teres to run on the interosseous membrane between and covered by flexor digitorum profundus and flexor pollicis longus ending beneath pronator quadratus.

Recurrent branch of median N. Runs out of the carpal tunnel over the distal border of the flexor retinaculum onto flexor pollicis brevis to terminate by passing into the thenar eminence.

6

6

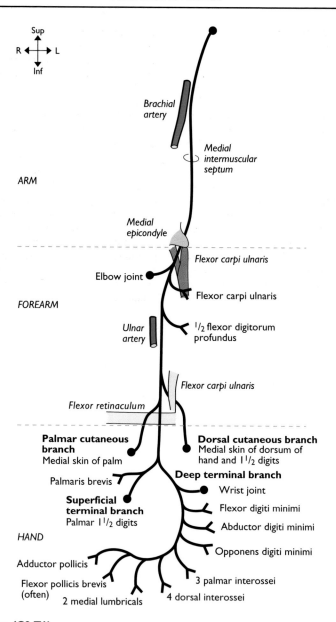

Sup

R ←┼→ L

Inf

ARM

Brachial
artery

Medial
intermuscular
septum

Medial
epicondyle

Elbow joint

FOREARM

Flexor carpi ulnaris

Flexor carpi ulnaris

Ulnar
artery

$1/2$ flexor digitorum
profundus

Flexor carpi ulnaris

Flexor retinaculum

**Palmar cutaneous
branch**
Medial skin of palm

Palmaris brevis

**Superficial
terminal branch**
Palmar $1^1/2$ digits

HAND

Adductor pollicis

Flexor pollicis brevis
(often)

2 medial lumbricals

Dorsal cutaneous branch
Medial skin of dorsum of
hand and $1^1/2$ digits

Deep terminal branch

Wrist joint

Flexor digiti minimi

Abductor digiti minimi

Opponens digiti minimi

3 palmar interossei

4 dorsal interossei

Ulnar nerve (C8,T1)

ULNAR NERVE (C8,T1)
From: Med cord of brachial plexus
To: Terminal brs

It arises medial to the axillary artery and continues medial to the brachial artery lying on coracobrachialis to the mid point of the humerus where it leaves the anterior compartment by passing posteriorly through the medial intermuscular septum with the superior ulnar collateral artery. It lies between the intermuscular septum and the medial head of triceps passing posterior to the medial humeral epicondyle and enters the forearm between the two heads of flexor carpi ulnaris. It then lies medial to the coronoid process of the ulna, runs deep to flexor carpi ulnaris and on flexor digitorum profundus, with the ulnar artery on its lateral side from one-third of the way down the forearm. It lies lateral to the tendon of flexor carpi ulnaris at the wrist and then passes superficial to the flexor retinaculum to divide into terminal branches at the pisiform bone.

Superficial terminal branch—lies superficial in the palm terminating as digital Ns. It also supplies palmaris brevis if present.

Deep terminal branch—passes through the hypothenar eminence between flexor digiti minimi and abductor digiti minimi grooving the hook of the hamate and runs with the deep palmar arch, deep to the flexor tendons to terminate in adductor pollicis.

Dorsal cutaneous branch—arises 5 cm proximal to the wrist, passes deep to flexor carpi ulnaris onto the medial aspect of the dorsum of the hand where it terminates as cutaneous Ns.

6

Phrenic nerve (C3,4,5)

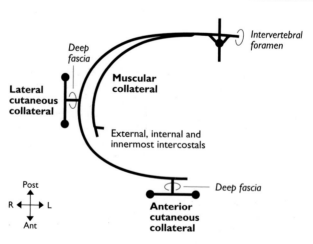

Intercostal nerve

PHRENIC NERVE (C3,4,5)
From: Ant primary rami of C3,4,5
To: Terminal brs

It arises deep between scalenus medius and scalenus anterior and runs over the lateral border of scalenus anterior behind the prevertebral fascia. It runs on scalenus anterior from lateral to medial edges lying lateral to the ascending cervical artery and it passes behind the suprascapular and transverse cervical arteries as it does so. It runs over the anterior part of the dome of the pleura to enter the mediastinum posterior to the subclavian vein and anterior to subclavian artery where right and left nerves take different courses. Right—spirals forwards to lie lateral to the right brachiocephalic vein and continues on the lateral surface of the superior vena cava, right atrium and inferior vena cava, lying within the fibrous pericardium. It passes anterior to the hilum of the lung before traversing the diaphragm via the caval orifice. Left—descends usually anterior to the left internal thoracic artery lying lateral to the left common carotid artery. It runs down over the aortic arch crossing anterior to the left vagus before running anterior to the left pulmonary artery and thus anterior to the hilum of the lung. It then runs lateral to the left auricle and left ventricle within the fibrous pericardium to traverse the diaphragm in isolation via the muscular portion of the diaphragm to the left of the central tendon.

An accessory phrenic N (C5) arising from the N to subclavius may join the phrenic N near the 1st rib.

INTERCOSTAL NERVE (TYPICAL)
From: Ant primary rami of thoracic N
To: Terminal brs

It emerges from the intervertebral foramen (giving off the posterior primary ramus as it does so) to pass between the pleura and the inner muscle layer anterior to the transverse process where it connects via the grey and white rami communicantes with the thoracic sympathetic chain. It passes posterior to the intercostal artery to lie below it as it runs in the subcostal groove in the plane between internal and innermost muscle layers. The muscular collateral branch arises before the posterior angle of the rib and runs in the same plane but lies at the level of the upper border of the rib below.

T1. Has no lateral or anterior cutaneous branches.

T7–11. Run behind the costal margins in their anterior course to lie in the same muscle plane in the abdomen. At their anterior limit they pass deep to rectus abdominis in the rectus sheath and pierce both of these structures to give terminal anterior cutaneous branches. These also supply rectus abdominis.

T12. Passes below the 12th rib as the subcostal N having similar branches to those above. It emerges from behind the lateral arcuate ligament of the diaphragm.

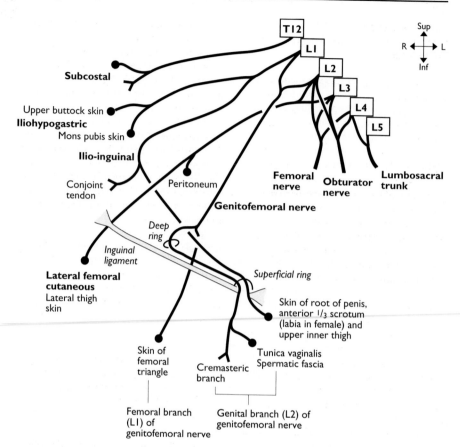

Lumbar plexus (T12,L1,2,3,4,5)

LUMBAR PLEXUS (T12,L1,2,3,4,5)
From: Ant primary rami of T12,L1,2,3,4,5
To: Ns as shown

The plexus is formed within the substance
of psoas major anterior to the transverse
processes of L2–5 from the anterior primary
rami as they emerge from the intervertebral
foramina.

Iliohypogastric N (L1). This main nerve
emerges lateral to psoas on the lumbar fascia
at the level of L2 to pass posterior to the
lower pole of the kidney and over quadratus
lumborum. It passes above the iliac crest,
between transversus and internal oblique
abdominis to pierce the latter above the
anterior superior iliac spine. It supplies both
muscles before becoming cutaneous.

Ilio-inguinal N (L1). This collateral branch
emerges lateral to psoas on the lumbar
fascia, passes posterior to the lower pole of
the kidney, over quadratus lumborum and
penetrates transversus and internal oblique
abdominis above the anterior superior iliac
spine. It supplies the lowest fibres of these
muscles and the conjoint tendon. Its terminal
branch enters the inguinal canal from above
to pass through the superficial inguinal ring
before piercing the external spermatic fascia
to become subcutaneous.

Lateral femoral cutaneous N (L2,3).
Emerges lateral to psoas below the iliac crest,
passes over iliacus obliquely lying posterior
to the caecum on the right and descending
colon on the left. It runs forward to the
anterior superior iliac spine where it
penetrates the inguinal ligament at its
attachment to pass into the subcutaneous
tissue of the lateral thigh.

Genitofemoral N (L1,2). Emerges onto the
anteromedial surface of psoas lying posterior
to the ureter, gonadal and iliocolic vessels on
the right and ureter, gonadal and lower left
colic vessels on the left. It divides into genital
and femoral branches on the anterior aspect
of psoas.

Genital branch. Crosses the external iliac
artery, passes through the deep inguinal ring
into the inguinal canal and through the
superficial inguinal ring to terminate in the
spermatic cord in the male and labium majus
in the female. It may also supply a small area
of scrotal/labial skin.

Femoral branch. Continues down lateral to
the external iliac artery, under the inguinal
ligament and into the femoral sheath which
it penetrates anteriorly to become
subcutaneous.

Lumbosacral trunk (L4,5). Emerges deep
from the medial aspect of psoas to pass over
the pelvic brim to form the upper fibres of
the sciatic N.

6

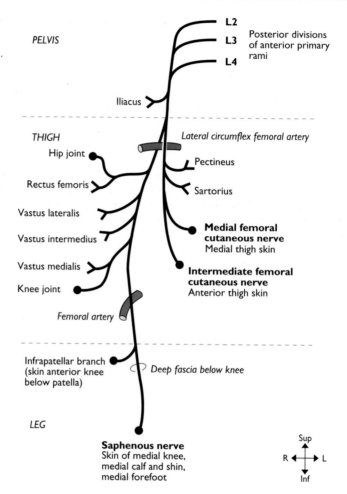

6

Femoral nerve (L2,3,4)

FEMORAL NERVE (L2,3,4)
From: **Post div of ant primary rami of L2,3,4**
To: **Terminal brs**

It is formed within psoas major and emerges from its lateral border low down in the iliac fossa to lie in the groove between psoas and iliacus. It reaches the thigh beneath the inguinal ligament lateral to the femoral artery lying on the tendon of iliacus and psoas. In the femoral triangle it splits into anterior and posterior divisions which straddle the lateral circumflex femoral artery. There are usually four short super- ficial branches. The deep branches continue down the femoral triangle, the N to vastus

medialis running lateral to the femoral artery as far as the upper part of the adductor (Hunter's) canal before entering the muscle.

Saphenous N (post division). Descends in the femoral triangle to reach the adductor canal where it spirals over the femoral artery to lie medial to it. It pierces the deep fascia through the apex of the canal and emerges posterior to sartorius and anterior to gracilis to continue with the long saphenous vein. It passes over the subcutaneous surface of the tibia and anterior to the medial malleolus where it is palpable, closely related to the long saphenous vein. It terminates in branches over the medial side of the foot.

6

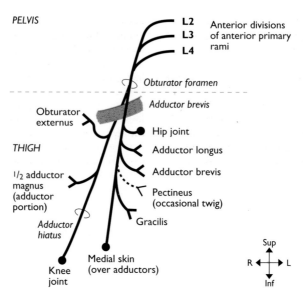

PELVIS

L2
L3
L4

Anterior divisions
of anterior primary
rami

Obturator foramen

Adductor brevis

Obturator
externus

Hip joint

THIGH

Adductor longus

Adductor brevis

$^1/_2$ adductor
magnus
(adductor
portion)

Pectineus
(occasional twig)

Adductor
hiatus

Gracilis

Sup

Knee
joint

Medial skin
(over adductors)

R ← → L

Inf

Obturator nerve (L2,3,4)

6

OBTURATOR NERVE (L2,3,4)
From: Ant div of ant primary rami of L2,3,4
To: Terminal brs

This nerve is formed within psoas major and emerges from the medial aspect of the muscle on the ala of the sacrum to pass behind the common iliac vessels. It runs over the pelvic brim on the lateral wall of the pelvis and over the upper fibres of obturator internus to pass through the upper anterior aspect of the obturator foramen. It divides into anterior and posterior divisions which straddle adductor brevis. The posterior division pierces a few fibres of obturator externus and runs deep to adductor brevis on adductor magnus. The anterior division runs on the anterior aspect of adductor brevis deep to pectineus and then deep to adductor longus to end by contributing, together with the saphenous and medial femoral cutaneous N, to the subsartorial plexus which supplies the skin over the medial thigh.

6

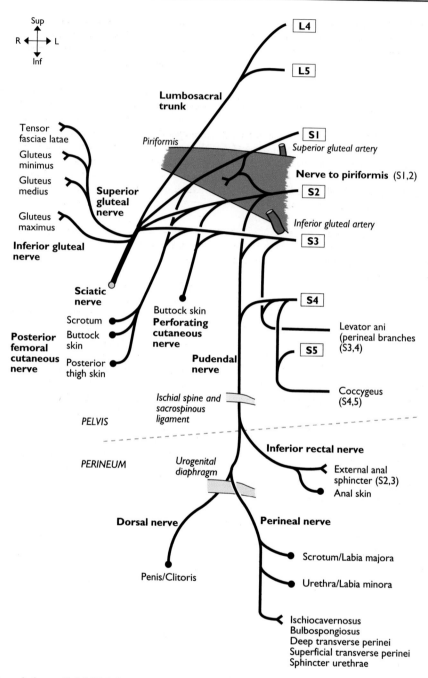

Sacral plexus (L4,5,S1,2,3,4,5)

SACRAL PLEXUS (L4,5,S1,2,3,4,5)

From: Lumbosacral trunk (L4,5) & ant
　primary rami from S1,2,3,4,5
To: Definitive Ns

Lies on piriformis on the posterior wall of
the pelvis deep to the internal iliac vessels
(and the sigmoid vessels on the left) and is
protected by a sheet of pelvic fascia overlying
it. Its roots are characteristically related to
arteries which pass between them as shown.

Superior gluteal N (L4,5,S1). Emerges from
the upper roots of the sciatic N and passes
out of the pelvis above piriformis through
the greater sciatic foramen. It runs between
gluteus medius and minimus over the middle
gluteal line on the outer surface of the ilium
to terminate in muscular branches.

Inferior gluteal N (L5,S1,2). Emerges from
the middle roots of the sciatic N and passes
out of the pelvis below piriformis through
the greater sciatic foramen to enter gluteus
maximus.

Posterior femoral cutaneous N (S1,2,3).
Passes out of the pelvis below piriformis
through the greater sciatic foramen. It runs
on the sciatic N, over the long head of biceps
femoris to become subcutaneous extending
as far as the popliteal fossa.

Perforating cutaneous N (S2,3). Passes
through the sacrotuberous ligament and
inferior to gluteus maximus to become subcutaneous in the buttock. It supplies that
part of the buttocks which touch when
standing and part when sitting.

Pudendal N (S2,3,4). Passes out of the pelvis
over the sacrospinous ligament close to the
ischial spine through the greater, and re-
entering through the lesser, sciatic foramina.
It runs on the medial surface of the lower
fibres of obturator internus in the pudendal
(Alcock's) canal. It passes forwards in the
lateral wall of the ischio-anal fossa where it
gives off its inferior rectal branch. It passes
into the perineum and gives its terminal
branches, the perineal N being superficial to
the urogenital diaphragm and the dorsal N
deep to it.

It helps to remember that all six branches
leaving sacral roots before anterior and
posterior divisions begin with the letter 'P':
N to Piriformis S1,2 (remains in pelvis to
　supply this muscle)
Posterior femoral cutaneous N S1,2,3 (leaves
　pelvis via greater sciatic foramen)
Perforating cutaneous N S2,3 (leaves pelvis
　via greater sciatic foramen)
Pudendal N S2,3,4 (leaves pelvis via greater
　sciatic foramen)
Pelvic splanchnics (parasympathetic) S2,3,4
　(remain in pelvis to supply pelvic organs)
Perineal branch of S4 (remains in pelvis to
　supply levator ani)

6

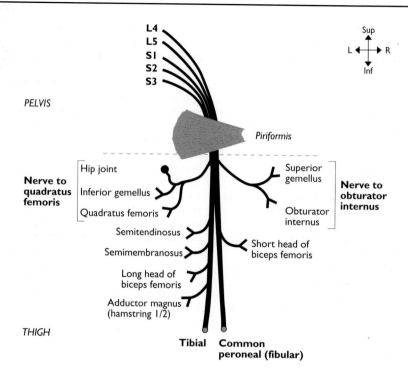

Sciatic nerve (L4,5,S1,2,3)

Viewed from behind

SCIATIC NERVE (L4,5,S1,2,3)
From: Ant primary rami of L4,5,S1,2,3
To: Tibial & common peroneal (fibular) Ns

It is formed in the upper sacral plexus and passes out of the greater sciatic foramen below piriformis. In the buttock and thigh it lies initially deep to gluteus maximus lying on gemellus superior, obturator internus tendon and gemellus inferior and then on quadratus femoris and adductor magnus. It passes out of the cover of gluteus maximus and for a short distance it is covered by only deep fascia, before it passes deep to the two heads of biceps femoris. It runs vertically down in the midline of the posterior compartment of the thigh and terminates by dividing into common peroneal (fibular) and tibial Ns usually two-thirds of the way down the thigh. In its course over the gemelli it is a close posterior relation of the ischium and posterior rim of the acetabulum.

N to quadratus femoris (L4,5,S1). Arises from the anterior surface of the sciatic N in the pelvis and leaves the pelvis in this position through the greater sciatic foramen, lying between the sciatic N and the ischium. Running deep to the tendon of obturator internus and the gemelli it supplies gemellus inferior before passing into quadratus femoris from above.

N to obturator internus (L5,S1,2). Arises from the anterior surface of the sciatic N in the pelvis and leaves the pelvis through the greater sciatic foramen below piriformis and medial to the sciatic N. It passes medially over the ischial spine (lateral to the pudendal neurovascular bundle) and sends a branch to gemellus superior before turning forward to pass through the lesser sciatic foramen, penetrating and supplying obturator internus as it does so.

6

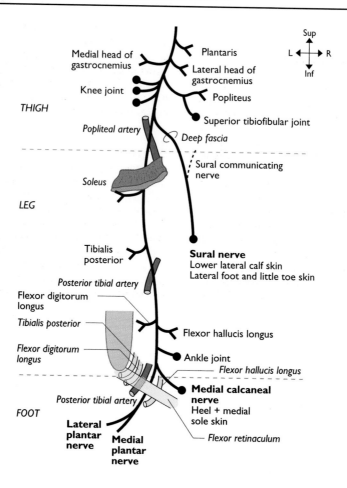

Sup

L ← → R

Inf

Plantaris

Medial head of gastrocnemius

Lateral head of gastrocnemius

Knee joint

Popliteus

THIGH

Superior tibiofibular joint

Popliteal artery

Deep fascia

Sural communicating nerve

Soleus

LEG

Tibialis posterior

Sural nerve
Lower lateral calf skin
Lateral foot and little toe skin

Posterior tibial artery

Flexor digitorum longus

Tibialis posterior

Flexor digitorum longus

Flexor hallucis longus

Ankle joint

Flexor hallucis longus

Posterior tibial artery

Medial calcaneal nerve
Heel + medial sole skin

FOOT

Lateral plantar nerve

Medial plantar nerve

Flexor retinaculum

Viewed from behind

Tibial nerve (L4,5,S1,2,3)

TIBIAL NERVE (L4,5,S1,2,3)
From: Sciatic N
To: Med & lat plantar Ns

It arises in the lower third of the thigh above the apex of the popliteal fossa as the larger terminal branch of the sciatic N, and passes down in the midline into the fossa between semitendinosus and biceps femoris, lying deep to them. It lies markedly lateral to the popliteal artery on entry to the popliteal fossa but then the artery crosses deep to the N to lie lateral to it. The tibial N and the popliteal artery remain separated by the popliteal veins. The nerve leaves the fossa deep to the two heads of gastrocnemius by passing deep to the fibrous arch of soleus. It then runs deep to soleus on tibialis posterior in the midline, crossing over the posterior tibial artery from medial to lateral half way down the calf. It slopes gently medially in the lower calf passing behind the medial malleolus of the lower tibia between the posterior tibial artery anteromedially and the tendon of flexor hallucis longus posterolaterally. It runs under the flexor retinaculum where it divides into terminal branches.

Sural N. Arises in the popliteal fossa, passing out posteriorly over the 'V' behind the two heads of gastrocnemius and is joined by the sural communicating N from the common peroneal (fibular) N. It pierces the deep fascia to become subcutaneous. It runs down laterally accompanied by the short saphenous vein to pass behind the lateral malleolus over the superior peroneal (fibular) retinaculum to end in terminal branches on the lateral side of the foot.

6

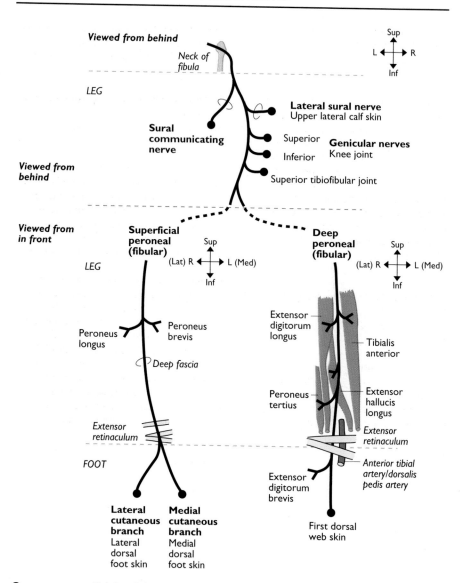

Common, superficial and deep peroneal (fibular) nerves
Note: the common peroneal (fibular) nerve is viewed from behind but the superficial and deep
nerves are viewed from in front

COMMON PERONEAL [FIBULAR] NERVE (L4,5,S1,2)
From: Sciatic N
To: Superficial & deep peroneal (fibular) Ns

It arises in the lower third of the thigh above the apex of the popliteal fossa as the smaller terminal branch of the sciatic N. It passes into the popliteal fossa along the upper lateral boundary just beneath the edge of biceps femoris and runs over plantaris, the lateral head of gastrocnemius and the posterior capsule of the knee joint. It runs over the fibular attachment of soleus to wind around the neck of the fibula from posterior to lateral. It passes into peroneus longus where it divides.

SUPERFICIAL PERONEAL [FIBULAR] NERVE (L5,S1,2)
From: Common peroneal (fibular) N
To: Terminal brs

It arises deep to peroneus longus and passes forwards and downwards to lie over the lateral surface of the fibula between peroneus longus and brevis. It pierces the deep fascia half way down the leg to become subcutaneous. It runs downwards superficial to the superior and inferior extensor retinacula to end as terminal branches over them.

DEEP PERONEAL [FIBULAR] NERVE (L4,5,S1,2)
From: Common peroneal (fibular) N
To: Terminal brs

It arises deep to peroneus longus and passes forwards deep to the muscle to wind around the fibula and to pass through the anterior intermuscular septum. It continues deep to extensor digitorum longus to appear between it and tibialis anterior lying on the interosseous membrane in the upper quarter of the anterior compartment. It runs down the interosseous membrane with the anterior tibial vessels, coming to lie between extensor hallucis longus and tibialis anterior in the lower three-quarters of the compartment. It passes anterior to the tibia at the ankle joint between the anterior tibial artery medially and the tendon of extensor digitorum longus laterally, running beneath the superior and inferior extensor retinacula. It breaks up into terminal branches on the dorsum of the foot. (Articular branch to ankle joint not shown.)

6

Lateral plantar nerve (S1,2)

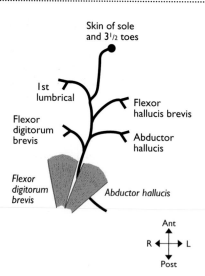

Medial plantar nerve (L4,5)

LATERAL PLANTAR NERVE (S1,2)
From: Tibial N
To: Terminal brs

It arises beneath the flexor retinaculum and runs forward with the lateral plantar artery around the sustentaculum tali of the calcaneus deep to abductor hallucis. It runs over the origin of flexor digitorum accessorius beneath flexor digitorum brevis, and its superficial terminal branches appear more superficially between flexor digitorum brevis and abductor digiti minimi. Its deep terminal branches run medially beneath the long flexor tendons and across the metatarsal shafts to end in muscular branches.

MEDIAL PLANTAR NERVE (L4,5)
From: Tibial N
To: Terminal brs

It arises beneath the flexor retinaculum and runs with the medial plantar artery around the sustentaculum tali of the calcaneus deep to abductor hallucis. It pierces the plantar fascia in so doing and runs forward over the tendon of flexor digitorum longus to appear more superficially again between abductor hallucis and flexor digitorum brevis in the sole of the foot.

6

Dermatomes: head and neck

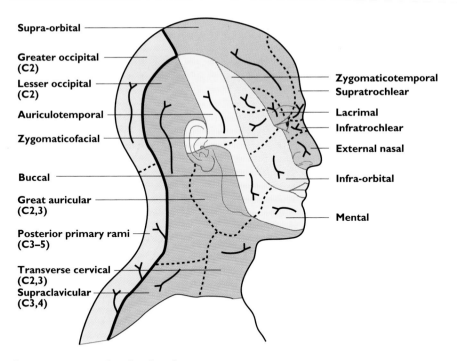

Supra-orbital

Greater occipital (C2)

Lesser occipital (C2)

Auriculotemporal

Zygomaticofacial

Buccal

Great auricular (C2,3)

Posterior primary rami (C3–5)

Transverse cervical (C2,3)

Supraclavicular (C3,4)

Zygomaticotemporal

Supratrochlear

Lacrimal

Infratrochlear

External nasal

Infra-orbital

Mental

Cutaneous nerves: head and neck

7

Dermatomes: upper limb

Cutaneous nerves: upper limb

Anterior

Posterior

Dermatomes: lower limb

7

Cutaneous nerves: lower limb

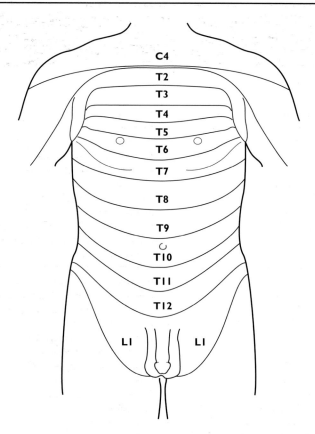

Dermatomes: thorax and abdomen

8

8

8

ABDUCTOR DIGITI MINIMI (foot)
Arises Med & lat processes of post calcaneal tuberosity
Inserts Lat side of base of prox phalanx of 5th toe & 5th MT
Action Flexes & abducts 5th toe. Supports lat longitudinal arch
Nerve Lat plantar N (S2,3)

ABDUCTOR DIGITI MINIMI (hand)
Arises Pisiform bone & pisohamate lig
Inserts Ulnar side of base of prox phalanx of little finger & extensor expansion (± sesamoid)
Action Abducts little finger at MCP jnt
Nerve Deep br of ulnar N (C8,T1)

ABDUCTOR HALLUCIS
Arises Med process of post calcaneal tuberosity & flexor retinaculum
Inserts Med aspect of base of prox phalanx of big toe via med sesamoid
Action Flexes & abducts big toe. Supports med longitudinal arch
Nerve Med plantar N (S1,2)

ABDUCTOR POLLICIS BREVIS
Arises Tubercle of scaphoid & flexor retinaculum
Inserts Radial sesamoid of prox phalanx of thumb & tendon of extensor pollicis longus
Action Abducts thumb at MCP & CMC jnts
Nerve Recurrent (muscular) br of median N (C8,T1)
Notes As this muscle is supplied only by median N, its action is used as a test for this N in hand

ABDUCTOR POLLICIS LONGUS
Arises Upper post surface of ulna & middle third of post surface of radius & interosseous membrane between
Inserts Over tendons of radial extensors & brachioradialis to base of 1st MC & trapezium

Action Abducts & extends thumb at CMC jnt
Nerve Post interosseous N (C7,8)
Notes Forms radial side of snuff box

ADDUCTOR BREVIS
Arises Inf ramus & body of pubis
Inserts Upper third of linea aspera
Action Adducts hip
Nerve Ant div of obturator N (L2,3)

ADDUCTOR HALLUCIS
Arises Oblique head: base of 2, 3, 4 MTs. Transverse head: plantar MT ligs & deep transverse lig
Inserts Lat side of base of prox phalanx of big toe & lat sesamoid
Action Adducts & flexes MTP jnt of big toe. Supports transverse arch
Nerve Deep br of lat plantar N (S2,3)
Notes If muscle fibres are attached to 1st MT it can be regarded as opponens hallucis

ADDUCTOR LONGUS
Arises Body of pubis inf & med to pubic tubercle
Inserts Lower two-thirds of med linea aspera
Action Adducts hip
Nerve Ant div of obturator N (L2,3,4)

ADDUCTOR MAGNUS
Arises Adductor portion: ischiopubic ramus. Hamstring portion: lower outer quadrant of post surface of ischial tuberosity
Inserts Adductor portion: lower gluteal line & linea aspera. Hamstring portion: adductor tubercle
Action Adductor portion: adducts hip. Hamstring portion: extends hip
Nerve Adductor portion: post div of obturator N (L2,3,4). Hamstring portion: tibial portion of sciatic (L4)

8

ADDUCTOR POLLICIS

Arises Oblique head: base of 2nd & 3rd MCs, trapezoid & capitate. Transverse head: palmar border & shaft of 3rd MC

Inserts Ulnar sesamoid then ulnar side of base of prox phalanx & tendon of extensor pollicis longus

Action Adducts CMC jnt of thumb

Nerve Deep br of ulnar N (C8,T1)

ANCONEUS

Arises Smooth surface at lower extremity of post aspect of lat epicondyle of humerus

Inserts Lat side of olecranon

Action Weak extensor of elbow. Moves (abducts) ulna in pronation

Nerve Radial N (C7,8)

ARTICULARIS CUBITI (subanconeus)

Arises Deep distal surface of med head of triceps

Inserts Post capsule of elbow jnt

Action Lifts capsule away from jnt

Nerve Radial (C6,7,8)

ARTICULARIS GENU

Arises Two slips from ant femur below vastus intermedius

Inserts Apex of suprapatellar bursa

Action Retracts bursa as knee extends

Nerve Post div of femoral N (L2,3,4)

ARYEPIGLOTTICUS

Arises Apex of arytenoid cartilage

Inserts Lat border of epiglottis

Action Aids closure of additus of larynx

Nerve Recurrent laryngeal br of vagus N (X)

Note It is an extension of oblique arytenoid

AURICULARIS

Arises Cartilage of auricle

Inserts Galeal aponeurosis

Action Adjusts position of ear

Nerve Temporal & posterior auricular brs of facial N (VII)

BICEPS BRACHII

Arises Long head: supraglenoid tubercle of scapula. Short head: coracoid process of scapula with coracobrachialis

Inserts Post border of bicipital tuberosity of radius (over bursa) & bicipital aponeurosis to deep fascia & subcutaneous ulna

Action Supinates forearm, flexes elbow, weakly flexes shoulder

Nerve Musculocutaneous N (C5,6) (from lat cord)

Notes Supinates most effectively when elbow flexed

BICEPS FEMORIS

Arises Long head: upper inner quadrant of post surface of ischial tuberosity. Short head: middle third of linea aspera, lat supracondylar ridge of femur

Inserts Styloid process of head of fibula, lat collateral lig & lat tibial condyle

Action Flexes & lat rotates knee. Long head extends hip

Nerve Long head: tibial portion of sciatic N. Short head: common peroneal portion of sciatic N (both L5,S1,2)

BRACHIALIS

Arises Ant lower half of humerus & med & lat intermuscular septa

Inserts Coronoid process & tuberosity of ulna

Action Flexes elbow

Nerve Musculocutaneous N (C5,6) (from lat cord). Also small supply from radial N (C7)

BRACHIORADIALIS

Arises Upper two-thirds of lat supracondylar ridge of humerus & lat intermuscular septum

Inserts Base of styloid process of radius

Action Flexes arm at elbow & brings forearm into midprone position

Nerve Radial N (C5,6)

Notes Overlies radial N & art as they lie on supinator

8

BUCCINATOR

Arises Ext alveolar margins of maxilla & mandible by molar teeth, to maxillary tubercle & pterygoid hamulus & post mylohyoid line respectively, then via pterygomandibular raphe between bones

Inserts Decussates at modiolus of mouth & interdigitates with opposite side

Action Aids mastication by emptying vestibule, tenses cheeks in blowing & whistling, aids closure of mouth

Nerve Buccal br of facial N (VII)

BULBOSPONGIOSUS

Arises Perineal body (& midline raphe over corpus spongiosum in male)

Inserts Superficial perineal membrane & dorsal penile/clitoral aponeurosis

Action Male: aids emptying of urine & ejaculate from urethra. Female: closes vaginal introitus

Nerve Perineal br of pudendal N (S2,3,4)

CONSTRICTOR OF PHARYNX—INFERIOR

Arises Cricopharyngeus: lat aspect of arch of cricoid cartilage. Thyropharyngeus: oblique line on laminar of thyroid cartilage & fibrous cricothyroid arch

Inserts Cricopharyngeus: continuous with muscle of opposite side, behind pharynx. Thyropharyngeus: lower pharyngeal raphe

Action Aids swallowing. Cricopharyngeus acts as upper oesophageal sphincter

Nerve Pharyngeal plexus (IX, X & sympathetic) via pharyngeal br of X with its motor fibres from cranial accessory (XI)

Notes Killian's dehiscence is between the two parts post

CONSTRICTOR OF PHARYNX—MIDDLE

Arises Lower third of stylohyoid lig, lesser cornu & sup border of greater cornu of hyoid bone

Inserts Middle portion of pharyngeal raphe

Action Aids swallowing

Nerve Pharyngeal plexus (IX, X & sympathetic) via pharyngeal br of X with its motor fibres from cranial accessory N (XI)

CONSTRICTOR OF PHARYNX—SUPERIOR

Arises Lower two-thirds of med pterygoid plate, pterygomandibular raphe & post end of mylohyoid line on mandible

Inserts Upper midline pharyngeal raphe & pharyngeal tubercle of occiput

Action Aids swallowing

Nerve Pharyngeal plexus (IX, X & sympathetic) via pharyngeal br of X with its motor fibres from cranial accessory (XI)

CORACOBRACHIALIS

Arises Coracoid process of scapula with biceps brachii

Inserts Middle third of med border of humerus

Action Flexes & weakly adducts arm

Nerve Musculocutaneous N (C5,6,7) (from lat cord)

Notes Ligament of Struthers as embryological 3rd head. Musculocutaneous N runs through muscle

CORRUGATOR SUPERCILII

Arises Med superciliary arch

Inserts Skin of med forehead

Action Wrinkles forehead

Nerve Temporal br of facial N (VII)

CREMASTER

Arises Lower border of internal oblique & transversus abdominis in inguinal canal

Inserts Loops around spermatic cord & tunica vaginalis & some fibres return to attach to pubic tubercle

Action Retracts testis

Nerve Sympathetic & somatic fibres in genital br (L2) of genitofemoral N (L1,2)

CRICOTHYROID

Arises Anterolateral aspect of cricoid cartilage

Inserts Inf cornu & lower laminar of thyroid cartilage

Action Lengthens & tenses vocal cords by tilting thyroid cartilage forwards

Nerve Ext br of sup laryngeal br of vagus N (X)

DARTOS

Arises Subcutaneous tissue of scrotum, superficial to superficial fascia (Colles)

Inserts Skin & midline fibrous septum of scrotum

Action Corrugates scrotal skin

Nerve Sympathetic fibres in genital br (L2) of genitofemoral N (L1,2)

DEEP TRANSVERSE PERINEI

Arises Med aspect of ischiopubic ramus & body of ischium within deep perineal pouch

Inserts Midline raphe & perineal body

Action Fixes perineal body & supports pelvic viscera

Nerve Perineal br of pudendal N (S2,3,4)

DELTOID

Arises Lat third of clavicle, acromion, spine of scapula to deltoid tubercle

Inserts Middle of lat surface of humerus (deltoid tuberosity)

Action Abducts arm, ant fibres flex & med rotate, post fibres extend & lat rotate

Nerve Axillary N (C5,6) (from post cord)

DEPRESSOR ANGULI ORIS

Arises Outer surface of mandible inf to mental foramen

Inserts Modiolus at angle of mouth

Action Depresses & draws angle of mouth laterally

Nerve Mandibular br of facial N (VII)

DEPRESSOR LABII INFERIORIS

Arises Outer surface of mandible inferomedial to mental foramen

Inserts Skin of lower lip

Action Depresses & draws lower lip laterally

Nerve Mandibular br of facial N (VII)

DIAPHRAGM

Arises Vertebral: crura from bodies of L1,2 (left), L1–3 (right), together giving median arcuate lig. Costal: med & lat arcuate ligs, inner aspect of lower six ribs and costal cartilages
Sternal: two slips from post aspect of xiphoid

Inserts Trefoil central tendon

Action Inspiration & assists in raising intra-abdominal pressure

Nerve Phrenic N (motor) (C3,4,5). Sensory: phrenic, intercostals (6–12) & upper two lumbar N roots

DIGASTRIC

Arises Ant belly: digastric fossa on post surface of symphysis menti. Post belly: base of med aspect of mastoid process

Inserts Fibrous loop to lesser cornu of hyoid bone

Action Elevates hyoid bone. Aids swallowing & depresses mandible

Nerve Ant belly: mylohyoid N (Vc). Post belly: facial N (VII) before it enters parotid gland

ERECTOR SPINAE— ILIOCOSTOCERVICALIS

Arises Post angles of ribs

Inserts Transverse processes above & below

Action Extends & lat flexes spine

Nerve Post primary rami

Notes Divided into iliocostalis—lumborum, thoracis & cervicalis

ERECTOR SPINAE—LONGISSIMUS

Arises Transverse processes

Inserts Transverse processes several levels above

8

Action Extends spine
Nerve Post primary rami
Notes Divided into longissimus—thoracis, cervicis & capitis

ERECTOR SPINAE—SPINALIS
Arises Spinous processes
Inserts Spinous processes six levels above
Action Lat flexion of spine
Nerve Post primary rami
Notes Divided into spinalis—thoracis, cervicis & capitis

EXTENSOR CARPI RADIALIS BREVIS
Arises Common extensor origin on ant aspect of lat epicondyle of humerus
Inserts Post base of 3rd MC
Action Extends & abducts hand at wrist
Nerve Post interosseous N (C7,8)

EXTENSOR CARPI RADIALIS LONGUS
Arises Lower third of lat supracondylar ridge of humerus & lat intermuscular septum
Inserts Post base of 2nd MC
Action Extends & abducts hand at wrist
Nerve Radial N (C6,7)

EXTENSOR CARPI ULNARIS
Arises Common extensor origin on ant aspect of lat epicondyle of humerus
Inserts Base of 5th MC via groove by ulnar styloid
Action Extends & adducts hand at wrist
Nerve Post interosseous N (C7,8)

EXTENSOR DIGITI MINIMI (hand)
Arises Common extensor origin on ant aspect of lat epicondyle of humerus
Inserts Extensor expansion of little finger—usually two tendons which are joined by a slip from extensor digitorum at MCP jnt
Action Extends all jnts of little finger
Nerve Post interosseous N (C7,8)

EXTENSOR DIGITORUM (hand)
Arises Common extensor origin on ant aspect of lat epicondyle of humerus
Inserts Extensor expansion to all phalanges of four fingers by four tendons. Tendons 3 & 4 usually fuse & little finger just receives a slip
Action Extends all jnts of fingers
Nerve Post interosseous N (C7,8)

EXTENSOR DIGITORUM BREVIS (foot)
Arises Sup surface of ant calcaneus
Inserts Four tendons into prox phalanx of big toe & long extensor tendons to toes 2, 3 and 4
Action Extends toes when foot fully dorsiflexed
Nerve Deep peroneal N (L5,S1)
Notes Med one of four tendons could be regarded as extensor hallucis brevis

EXTENSOR DIGITORUM LONGUS (foot)
Arises Upper two-thirds of ant shaft of fibula, interosseous membrane & sup tibiofibular jnt
Inserts Extensor expansion of lat four toes
Action Extends toes & extends foot at ankle
Nerve Deep peroneal N (L5,S1)

EXTENSOR HALLUCIS LONGUS
Arises Middle half of ant shaft of fibula
Inserts Dorsal base of distal phalanx of great toe
Action Extends big toe & foot. Inverts foot & tightens subtalar jnts
Nerve Deep peroneal N (L5,S1)

EXTENSOR INDICIS
Arises Lower post shaft of ulna (below extensor pollicis longus) & adjacent interosseous membrane
Inserts Extensor expansion of index finger (tendon lies on ulnar side of extensor digitorum tendon)

Action Extends all jnts of index finger

Nerve Post interosseous N (C7,8)

EXTENSOR POLLICIS BREVIS

Arises Lower third of post shaft of radius & adjacent interosseous membrane

Inserts Over tendons of radial extensors & brachioradialis to base of prox phalanx of thumb

Action Extends MCP jnt of thumb

Nerve Post interosseous N (C7,8)

Notes Forms radial side of snuff box

EXTENSOR POLLICIS LONGUS

Arises Middle third of post ulna (below abductor pollicis longus) & adjacent interosseous membrane

Inserts Base of distal phalanx of thumb via Lister's tubercle (dorsal tubercle of radius)

Action Extends IP & MCP jnts of thumb

Nerve Post interosseous N (C7,8)

Notes Forms ulnar side of snuff box

EXTERNAL OBLIQUE ABDOMINIS

Arises Ant angles of lower eight ribs

Inserts Outer ant half of iliac crest, inguinal lig, pubic tubercle & crest, & aponeurosis of ant rectus sheath, linea alba & xiphisternum

Action Supports abdominal wall, assists forced expiration, aids raising intra-abdominal pressure &, with muscles of opposite side, abducts & rotates trunk

Nerve Ant primary rami (T7–12)

Notes Interdigitates with four slips of serratus anterior & four of latissimus dorsi

FLEXOR CARPI RADIALIS

Arises Common flexor origin of med epicondyle of humerus

Inserts Bases of 2nd & 3rd MCs via groove in trapezium

Action Flexes & abducts wrist

Nerve Median N (C6,7) (from med & lat cords)

FLEXOR CARPI ULNARIS

Arises Humeral head: common flexor origin of med epicondyle. Ulnar head: aponeurosis from med olecranon & upper three-quarters subcutaneous border of ulna

Inserts Pisiform, hook of hamate, base of 5th MC via pisohamate & pisometacarpal ligs

Action Flexes & adducts wrist. Fixes pisiform during action of hypothenar muscles

Nerve Ulnar N (C7,8,T1) (by communication from lat cord)

Notes Ulnar N passes between two heads

FLEXOR DIGITI MINIMI BREVIS (foot)

Arises Base of 5th MT & sheath of peroneus longus

Inserts Lat side of base of prox phalanx of little toe

Action Flexes MTP jnt of little toe

Nerve Superficial br of lat plantar N (S2,3)

Notes A few muscle fibres to distal half of plantar surface of 5th MT represent opponens digiti minimi

FLEXOR DIGITI MINIMI BREVIS (hand)

Arises Flexor retinaculum & hook of hamate

Inserts Ulnar side of base of prox phalanx of little finger

Action Flexes MCP jnt of little finger

Nerve Deep br of ulnar N (C8,T1)

FLEXOR DIGITORUM ACCESSORIUS (QUADRATUS PLANTAE) (foot)

Arises Med & lat sides of calcaneus

Inserts Tendons of flexor digitorum longus

Action Assists flexor digitorum longus to flex lat four toes, especially when ankle is plantar flexed

Nerve Lat plantar N (S2,3)

FLEXOR DIGITORUM BREVIS (foot)

Arises Med process of post calcaneal tuberosity

8

Inserts Four tendons to four lat toes to both sides of middle phalanx. Tendons of flexor digitorum longus pass through them

Action Flexes lat four toes. Supports med & lat longitudinal arches

Nerve Med plantar N (S1,2)

FLEXOR DIGITORUM LONGUS (foot)

Arises Post shaft of tibia below soleal line & by broad aponeurosis from fibula

Inserts Base of distal phalanges of lat four toes

Action Flexes distal phalanges of lat four toes & foot at ankle. Supports lat longitudinal arch

Nerve Tibial N (S2,3)

Notes Med two tendons receive slips from flexor hallucis longus & all four receive insertion of flexor accessorius & each gives a lumbrical

FLEXOR DIGITORUM
PROFUNDUS (hand)

Arises Upper three-quarters of ant & med surface of ulna as far round as subcutaneous border & narrow strip of interosseous membrane

Inserts Distal phalanges of med four fingers. Tendon to index finger separates early

Action Flexes distal IP jnts, then secondarily flexes prox IP & MCP jnts & wrist

Nerve Median N (ant interosseous) (C8,T1) ulnar N (C8,T1)

Notes Nerve supply as above in 60%. In 40% it is a 3:1 ratio either way

FLEXOR DIGITORUM
SUPERFICIALIS (hand)

Arises Humeral head: common flexor origin of med epicondyle of humerus, med lig of elbow. Ulnar head: sublime tubercle (med border of coronoid process) & fibrous arch. Radial head: whole length of ant oblique line

Inserts Tendons split to insert onto sides of middle phalanges of med four fingers

Action Flexes prox IP jnts & secondarily MCP jnts & wrist

Nerve Median N (C7,8,T1) (from med & lat cords)

Notes Median N applied to under surface of muscle

FLEXOR HALLUCIS BREVIS

Arises Cuboid, lat cuneiform & tibialis posterior insertion over the two remaining cuneiforms

Inserts Med tendon to med side of base of prox phalanx of big toe. Lat tendon to lat side of same, both via sesamoids

Action Flexes MTP jnt of big toe. Supports med longitudinal arch

Nerve Med plantar N (S1,2)

FLEXOR HALLUCIS LONGUS

Arises Lower two-thirds of post fibula between median crest & post border, lower intermuscular septum & interosseous membrane

Inserts Base of distal phalanx of big toe & slips to med two tendons of flexor digitorum longus

Action Flexes distal phalanx of big toe, flexes foot at ankle, supports med logitudinal arch

Nerve Tibial N (S2,3)

FLEXOR POLLICIS BREVIS

Arises Superficial head: flexor retinaculum & tubercle of trapezium. Deep head: capitate & trapezoid

Inserts Base of prox phalanx of thumb (via radial sesamoid)

Action Flexes MCP jnt of thumb

Nerve Recurrent (muscular) br of median N (C8,T1) (may also be from deep br of ulnar N (C8,T1))

FLEXOR POLLICIS LONGUS

Arises Ant surface of radius below ant oblique line & adjacent interosseous membrane

Inserts Base of distal phalanx of thumb

8

Action Flexes distal phalanx of thumb
Nerve Ant interosseous N (C7,8)

GASTROCNEMIUS
Arises Lat head: post surface of lat condyle
of femur & highest of three facets on lat
condyle. Med head: post surface of femur
above med condyle
Inserts Tendo calcaneus to middle of three
facets on post aspect of calcaneus
Action Plantar flexes foot. Flexes knee
Nerve Tibial N (S1,2)
Notes Main propulsive force for jumping

GEMELLUS INFERIOR
Arises Upper border of ischial tuberosity
Inserts Middle part of med aspect of greater
trochanter of femur
Action Lat rotates & stabilises hip
Nerve N to quadratus femoris (L4,5,S1)

GEMELLUS SUPERIOR
Arises Spine of ischium
Inserts Middle part of med aspect of greater
trochanter of femur
Action Lat rotates & stabilises hip
Nerve N to obturator internus (L5,S1,2)

GENIOGLOSSUS
Arises Sup mental spine on post surface of
symphysis menti
Inserts Central mass of tongue & mucous
membrane
Action Protracts tongue
Nerve Hypoglossal N (XII)

GENIOHYOID
Arises Inf mental spine on post surface of
symphysis menti
Inserts Sup border of body of hyoid bone
Action Elevates & protracts hyoid bone.
Depresses mandible
Nerve C1 fibres carried by hypoglossal N
(XII)

GLUTEUS MAXIMUS
Arises Outer surface of ilium behind post
gluteal line & post third of iliac crest,
lumbar fascia, lat mass of sacrum,
sacrotuberous lig & coccyx
Inserts Deepest quarter into gluteal
tuberosity of femur, remaining three-
quarters into iliotibial tract (ant surface of
lat condyle of tibia)
Action Extends & lat rotates hip.
Maintains knee extended via iliotibial
tract
Nerve Inf gluteal N (L5,S1,2)
Notes Largest muscle in body

GLUTEUS MEDIUS
Arises Outer surface of ilium between post
& ant gluteal lines
Inserts Posterolateral surface of greater
trochanter of femur
Action Abducts & med rotates hip. Tilts
pelvis on walking
Nerve Sup gluteal N (L4,5,S1)

GLUTEUS MINIMUS
Arises Outer surface of ilium between ant
& inf gluteal lines
Inserts Ant surface of greater trochanter of
femur
Action Abducts & med rotates hip. Tilts
pelvis on walking
Nerve Sup gluteal N (L4,5,S1)

GRACILIS
Arises Outer surface of ischiopubic
ramus
Inserts Upper med shaft of tibia behind
sartorius
Action Adducts hip. Flexes knee & med
rotates flexed knee
Nerve Ant div of obturator N (L2,3)

HYOGLOSSUS
(& CHONDROGLOSSUS)
Arises Sup border of greater cornu of hyoid
bone
Inserts Lat side of tongue

8

Action Depresses tongue
Nerve Hypoglossal N (XII)

ILIACUS
Arises Iliac fossa within abdomen
Inserts Lowermost surface of lesser
trochanter of femur
Action Flexes hip
Nerve Femoral N in abdomen (L2,3)

INFERIOR OBLIQUE (see also obliquus capitis inferior)
Arises Orbital surface of maxilla behind
orbital margin on med side
Inserts Post/inf quadrant of sclera behind
equator of eyeball on lat side
Action Elevates eye in adduction. Extorts
eye in abduction
Nerve Inf div of oculomotor N (III)

INFERIOR RECTUS
Arises Inf tendinous ring within orbit
Inserts Inf sclera ant to equator of eyeball
Action Depresses eye. Extorts eye in
adduction
Nerve Inf div of oculomotor N (III)

INFRASPINATUS
Arises Med three-quarters of infraspinous
fossa of scapula & fibrous intermuscular
septa
Inserts Middle facet of greater tuberosity
of humerus & capsule of shoulder jnt
Action Lat rotates arm & stabilises
shoulder jnt
Nerve Suprascapular N (C5,6) (from upper
trunk)
Notes Bursa under tendon over glenoid
angle. Tendon forms part of rotator cuff

INTERCOSTALS EXTERNAL
Arises Inf border of ribs as far forwards as
costochondral junctions. Beyond this is
ant (ext) intercostal membrane
Inserts Sup border of ribs below, passing
obliquely downwards & forwards

Action Fix intercostal spaces during
respiration. Aids forced respiration by
elevating ribs
Nerve Muscular collateral brs of intercostal
Ns

INTERCOSTALS INNERMOST
Arises Int lat aspect of ribs above & below
Inserts Int aspect of ribs above & below
Action Fix intercostal spaces during
respiration
Nerve Muscular collateral brs of intercostal
Ns
Notes Innermost intercostals are one of
three muscles that make up inner layer
of thoracic wall muscles. Others are
transversus thoracis (ant) & subcostalis
(post)

INTERCOSTALS INTERNAL
Arises Inf border of ribs as far back as post
angles. Beyond this is post (int) intercostal
membrane
Inserts Sup border of ribs below, passing
obliquely downwards & backwards
Action Fix intercostal spaces during
respiration. Aids forced inspiration by
elevating ribs
Nerve Muscular collateral brs of intercostal
Ns

INTERNAL OBLIQUE ABDOMINIS
Arises Lumbar fascia, ant two-thirds of
iliac crest & lat two-thirds of inguinal lig
Inserts Costal margin (ribs & costal
cartilages), aponeurosis of rectus sheath
(ant & post), conjoint tendon to pubic
crest & pectineal line
Action Supports abdominal wall, assists
forced respiration, aids raising intra-
abdominal pressure &, with muscles of
other side, abducts & rotates trunk.
Conjoint tendon supports post wall of
inguinal canal
Nerve Ant primary rami (T7–12) (conjoint
tendon ilio-inguinal N (L1))

INTEROSSEI—DORSAL OF FOOT (4)
Arises Bipennate from inner aspects of shafts of all MTs
Inserts Bases of prox phalanges & dorsal extensor expansions of med side of 2nd toe & lat sides of 2nd, 3rd & 4th toes
Action Abduct 2nd, 3rd & 4th toes from axis of 2nd toe. Assist lumbricals in extending IP jnts whilst flexing MTP jnts
Nerve Lat plantar N (1–3: deep br; 4: superficial br) (S2,3)

INTEROSSEI—DORSAL OF HAND (4)
Arises Bipennate from inner aspects of shafts of all MCs
Inserts Prox phalanges & dorsal extensor expansion on radial side of index & middle fingers & ulnar side of middle & ring fingers
Action Abduct index, middle & ring fingers from axis of middle finger. Flex MCP jnt whilst extending IP jnts
Nerve Deep br of ulnar N (C8,T1)

INTEROSSEI—PALMAR OF HAND (3)
Arises Ant shafts of 2, 4, 5 MCs (unipennate)
Inserts Prox phalanges & dorsal extensor expansion on ulnar side of index & radial side of ring & little fingers
Action Adduct index, ring & little fingers to axis of middle finger. Flex MCP jnt whilst extending IP jnts
Nerve Deep br of ulnar N (C8,T1)

INTEROSSEI—PLANTAR OF FOOT (3)
Arises Inferomedial shafts of 3rd, 4th & 5th MTs (single heads)
Inserts Med sides of bases of prox phalanges with slips to dorsal extensor expansions of 3rd, 4th & 5th toes
Action Adduct 3rd, 4th & 5th toes to axis of 2nd toe. Assist lumbricals in extending IP jnts whilst flexing MTP jnts
Nerve Deep br of lat plantar N (S2,3)

INTERSPINALES
Arises Spinous processes
Inserts Spinous processes one above
Action Extension of spine
Nerve Post primary rami

INTERTRANSVERSARII
Arises Transverse processes
Inserts Transverse processes one above
Action Lat flexes spine
Nerve Post primary rami

INTRINSIC MUSCLE OF TONGUE
Arises Sup & inf longitudinal, transverse & vertical elements
Inserts Mucous membrane, septum & other muscles of tongue
Action Alter shape of tongue & so aid mastication, speech & swallowing
Nerve Hypoglossal N (XII)

ISCHIOCAVERNOSUS
Arises Med aspect of ischium & ischiopubic ramus
Inserts Inferolateral aponeurosis over crura of penis/clitoris
Action Stabilises erect penis
Nerve Perineal br of pudendal N (S2,3,4)

8

LATERAL CRICOARYTENOID
Arises Lat aspect of arch of cricoid cartilage
Inserts Muscular process of arytenoid cartilage
Action Adducts & med rotates arytenoid cartilage (closes rima glottidis)
Nerve Recurrent laryngeal br of vagus N (X)

LATERAL PTERYGOID
Arises Upper head: infratemporal surface of sphenoid bone. Lower head: lat surface of lat pterygoid plate
Inserts Pterygoid fovea below condylar process of mandible & intra-articular disc & capsule of temporomandibular jnt
Action Protrudes mandible & opens mouth by pulling condyle & disc forwards
Nerve Ns to lat pterygoid (ant div of mandibular N (Vc))

LATERAL RECTUS
Arises Lat tendinous ring within orbit
Inserts Lat sclera ant to equator of eyeball
Action Abducts eye
Nerve Abducent N (VI)

LATISSIMUS DORSI
Arises All thoracic spines & supraspinous ligs from T7 downwards & lumbar & sacral spines via lumbar fascia, post third iliac crest, last four ribs (interdigitating with ext oblique abdominis) & inf angle of scapula
Inserts Floor of bicipital groove of humerus after spiraling around teres major
Action Extends, adducts & med rotates arm. Costal attachment helps with deep inspiration & forced expiration
Nerve Thoracodorsal N (C6,7,8) (from post cord)

LEVATOR ANGULI ORIS
Arises Ant surface of maxilla below infraorbital foramen
Inserts Outer end of upper lip & modiolus
Action Elevates angle of mouth
Nerve Buccal br of facial N (VII)

LEVATOR ANI—COCCYGEUS
Arises Sacrospinous lig & ischial spine
Inserts Anococcygeal body & coccyx
Action Supports pelvic viscera
Nerve Ant primary rami (perineal brs) of S4,5

LEVATOR ANI—ILIOCOCCYGEUS
Arises Post half of fascial line over obturator internus & ischial spine
Inserts Anococcygeal body
Action Supports pelvic viscera
Nerve Ant primary rami (perineal brs) of S3,4

LEVATOR ANI—PUBOCOCCYGEUS
Arises Post surface of pubis & ant half of fascial line over obturator internus
Inserts Anococcygeal body
Action Supports pelvic viscera
Nerve Ant primary rami (perineal brs) of S3,4

LEVATOR ANI—PUBORECTALIS
Arises Post surface of pubis
Inserts Midline sling post to rectum
Action Supports & aids continence of rectum by maintaining anorectal angle
Nerve Ant primary rami (perineal brs) of S3,4

LEVATOR ANI—PUBOVAGINALIS (LEVATOR PROSTATAE)
Arises Post surface of pubis
Inserts Midline raphe post to vagina/prostate
Action Supports ant pelvic viscera
Nerve Ant primary rami (perineal brs) of S3,4

LEVATOR LABII SUPERIORIS
Arises Med infra-orbital margin
Inserts Skin & muscle of upper lip
Action Elevates & everts upper lip
Nerve Buccal br of facial N (VII)

LEVATOR LABII SUPERIORIS ALAEQUE NASI
Arises Upper frontal process of maxilla
Inserts Skin of lat nostril & upper lip
Action Dilates nostril & elevates upper lip
Nerve Buccal br of facial N (VII)

LEVATOR PALPEBRAE SUPERIORIS
Arises Inf aspect of lesser wing of sphenoid bone just above tendinous ring
Inserts Sup tarsal plate & skin of upper eyelid
Action Elevates & retracts upper eyelid
Nerve Sup div of oculomotor N (III) & sympathetic to smooth muscle portion

8

LEVATOR SCAPULAE
Arises Post tubercles of transverse processes of C1–4
Inserts Upper part of med border of scapula
Action Raises med border of scapula
Nerve Ant primary rami of C3 & C4 & dorsal scapular N (C5)

LEVATOR VELI PALATINI
Arises Within pharynx at apex of inf surface of petrous temporal bone & med rim of auditory tube
Inserts Palatine aponeurosis
Action Elevates, retracts & lat deviates soft palate. May open auditory tube on swallowing
Nerve Pharyngeal plexus (IX, X, sympathetic) via pharyngeal br of vagus N (X) with its motor fibres from cranial accessory N (XI)

LEVATORES COSTARUM
Arises Transverse processes C7 to T11
Inserts Post surface & angle of rib below
Action Elevates ribs
Nerve Post primary rami

LONGUS CAPITIS
Arises Ant tubercles of transverse processes of C3–6
Inserts Ant basilar occipital bone
Action Flexes cervical spine & atlanto-occipital jnt
Nerve Ant primary rami of C1–3

LONGUS COLLI
Arises Ant body of T1–3, ant tubercles of transverse processes of C3–7
Inserts Ant arch of atlas (C1) & bodies of C2–4
Action Flexes & rotates cervical spine
Nerve Ant primary rami of C2–6

LUMBRICALS OF FOOT (4)
Arises Lat 3: bipennate origin from cleft between the four tendons of flexor digitorum longus. Med 1: unipennate origin from med aspect of 1st tendon
Inserts Dorsal extensor expansion
Action Extend toes at IP jnts & flex MTP jnts
Nerve First: med plantar N (S2,3). 2–4: deep br of lat plantar N (S2,3)

LUMBRICALS OF HAND (4)
Arises Four tendons of flexor digitorum profundus. Radial 2: radial side only (unipennate). Ulnar 2: cleft between tendons (bipennate)
Inserts Extensor expansion (dorsum of prox phalanx) of fingers 2–5 radial side
Action Flex MCP jnts & extend IP jnts of fingers
Nerve Lat 2: median N (C8,T1). Med 2: deep br of ulnar N (C8,T1)
Notes 60% have nerve supply as above. 40% have 3:1 or 1:3

MASSETER
Arises Ant two-thirds of zygomatic arch & zygomatic process of maxilla
Inserts Lat surface of angle & lower ramus of mandible
Action Elevates mandible (enables forced closure of mouth)
Nerve Ant div of mandibular N (Vc)

MEDIAL PTERYGOID
Arises Deep head. Med side of lat pterygoid plate & fossa between med & lat plates. Superficial head: tuberosity of maxilla & pyramidal process of palatine bone
Inserts Med aspect of angle of mandible
Action Elevates, protracts & lat displaces mandible to opposite side for chewing
Nerve N to medial pterygoid (main trunk of mandibular N (Vc))

MEDIAL RECTUS
Arises Med tendinous ring within orbit
Inserts Med sclera ant to equator of eyeball
Action Adducts eye
Nerve Inf div of oculomotor N (III)

8

MENTALIS
Arises Incisive fossa on ant aspect of mandible
Inserts Skin of chin
Action Elevates & wrinkles skin of chin & protrudes lower lip
Nerve Mandibular br of facial N (VII)

MUSCULUS UVULAE
Arises Post border of hard palate
Inserts Palatine aponeurosis
Action Shapes uvula
Nerve Pharyngeal plexus (IX, X, sympathetic) via pharyngeal br of vagus N (X) with its motor fibres from cranial accessory N (XI)

MYLOHYOID
Arises Mylohyoid line on int aspect of mandible
Inserts Ant three-quarters: midline raphe. Post quarter: sup border of body of hyoid bone
Action Elevates hyoid bone, supports & raises floor of mouth. Aids in mastication & swallowing
Nerve Mylohyoid N (Vc)

NASALIS (COMPRESSOR & DILATOR)
Arises Frontal process of maxilla
Inserts Nasal aponeurosis
Action Opens & closes nostrils, particularly in forced respiration
Nerve Buccal br of facial N (VII)
Notes Part of dilator nasalis is depressor septi from maxilla above central incisor to mobile part of nasal septum

OBLIQUE ARYTENOID
Arises Muscular process of arytenoid cartilage
Inserts Sup pole of opposite arytenoid cartilage
Action Adducts arytenoid cartilages (closes rima glottidis)

Nerve Recurrent laryngeal br of vagus N (X)
Notex It extends into aryepiglottic fold as aryepiglotticus

OBLIQUUS CAPITIS INFERIOR
Arises Spinous process of axis (C2)
Inserts Lat mass of atlas (C1)
Action Rotates atlanto-axial jnt
Nerve Suboccipital N (post primary ramus of C1)

OBLIQUUS CAPITIS SUPERIOR
Arises Lat mass of atlas (C1)
Inserts Lat half inf nuchal line
Action Lat flexes atlanto-occipital jnt
Nerve Suboccipital N (post primary ramus of C1)

OBTURATOR EXTERNUS
Arises Outer obturator membrane, rim of pubis & ischium bordering it
Inserts Trochanteric fossa on med surface of greater trochanter
Action Lat rotates hip
Nerve Post div of obturator N (L3,4)

OBTURATOR INTERNUS
Arises Inner surface of obturator membrane & rim of pubis & ischium bordering membrane
Inserts Middle part of med aspect of greater trochanter of femur
Action Lat rotates & stabilises hip
Nerve N to obturator internus (L5,S1,2)

OCCIPITOFRONTALIS
Arises Occipital: highest nuchal line & mastoid process. Frontal: sup fibres of upper facial muscles
Inserts Galeal aponeurosis
Action Wrinkles forehead & fixes galeal aponeurosis
Nerve Post auricular & temporal brs of facial N (VII)

OMOHYOID
Arises Suprascapular lig & adjacent scapula
Inserts Inf border of body of hyoid bone
Action Depresses hyoid bone & hence larynx
Nerve Ansa cervicalis N (C1,2,3)
Notes Tendon between two bellies through sling behind sternocleidomastoid

OPPONENS DIGITI MINIMI (hand)
Arises Flexor retinaculum & hook of hamate
Inserts Ulnar border of shaft of 5th MC
Action Opposes (flexes & lat rotates) CMC jnt of little finger
Nerve Deep br of ulnar N (C8,T1)

OPPONENS POLLICIS
Arises Flexor retinaculum & tubercle of trapezium
Inserts Whole of radial border of 1st MC
Action Opposes (med rotates & flexes) CMC jnt of thumb
Nerve Recurrent (muscular) br of median N (C8,T1) (may also be from deep br of ulnar N (C8,T1))

ORBICULARIS OCULI
Arises Med orbital margin & lacrimal fascia behind lacrimal sac (orbital, palpebral & lacrimal parts)
Inserts Lat palpebral raphe
Action Closes eyelids, aids passage & drainage of tears
Nerve Temporal & zygomatic brs of facial N (VII)

ORBICULARIS ORIS
Arises Near midline on ant surface of maxilla & mandible & modiolus at angle of mouth
Inserts Mucous membrane of margin of lips & raphe with buccinator at modiolus
Action Narrows orifice of mouth, purses lips & puckers lip edges
Nerve Buccal br of facial N (VII)

Notes Accessory parts are incisivus labii superioris & inferioris

PALATOGLOSSUS
Arises Palatine aponeurosis
Inserts Posterolateral tongue
Action Elevates post tongue & closes oropharyngeal isthmus & aids initiation of swallowing
Nerve Pharyngeal plexus (IX, X, sympathetic) via pharyngeal br of vagus N (X) with its motor fibres from cranial accessory N (XI)
Notes Forms palatoglossal arch

PALATOPHARYNGEUS
Arises Palatine aponeurosis & post margin of hard palate
Inserts Upper border of thyroid cartilage & blends with constrictor fibres. Upper fibres interdigitate with opposite side to give Passavant's ridge
Action Elevates pharynx & larynx. Passavant's muscle closes nasopharyngeal isthmus in swallowing
Nerve Pharyngeal plexus (IX, X, sympathetic) via pharyngeal br of vagus N (X) with its motor fibres from cranial accessory N (XI)
Notes Forms palatoglopharyngeal arch

PALMARIS BREVIS
Arises Flexor retinaculum & palmar aponeurosis
Inserts Skin of palm into dermis
Action Steadies & corrugates skin of palm to help with grip
Nerve Superficial br of ulnar N (C8,T1)
Notes Only muscle supplied by this br of ulnar N

PALMARIS LONGUS
Arises Common flexor origin of med epicondyle of humerus
Inserts Flexor retinaculum & palmar aponeurosis

8

Action Flexes wrist & tenses palmar aponeurosis
Nerve Median N (C7,8) (from med & lat cords)
Notes Absent in 13%

PECTINEUS
Arises Pectineal line of pubis & narrow area of sup pubic ramus below it
Inserts A vertical line between spiral line & gluteal crest below lesser trochanter of femur
Action Flexes & adducts hip
Nerve Ant div of femoral N (L2,3). Occasional twig from obturator N (ant div—L2,3)

PECTORALIS MAJOR
Arises Clavicular head—med half clavicle. Sternocostal head—lat manubrium & sternum, six upper costal cartilages & ext oblique aponeurosis
Inserts Lat lip of bicipital groove of humerus and ant lip of deltoid tuberosity
Action Clavicular head: flexes & adducts arm. Sternal head: adducts & med rotates arm. Accessory for inspiration
Nerve Med pectoral N (from med cord) & lat pectoral N (from lat cord) (C6,7,8)
Notes Muscle folds on itself so that clavicular fibres insert lowest. Sternal fibres are highest inserting into capsule of shoulder joint

PECTORALIS MINOR
Arises Ant aspect of 3, 4, 5 ribs
Inserts Med & upper surface of coracoid process of scapula
Action Elevates ribs if scapula fixed, protracts scapula (assists serratus anterior)
Nerve Med & lat pectoral Ns (C6,7,8) (from med & lat cords)
Notes Landmark for axillary art & cords of brachial plexus

PERONEUS BREVIS
Arises Lower two-thirds lat shaft of fibula
Inserts Tuberosity of base of 5th MT
Action Plantar flexes & everts foot. Supports lat longitudinal arch
Nerve Superficial peroneal N (L5,S1)

PERONEUS LONGUS
Arises Upper two-thirds of lat shaft of fibula, head of fibula & sup tibiofibular jnt
Inserts Plantar aspect of base of 1st MT & med cuneiform, passing deep to long plantar lig
Action Plantar flexes & everts foot. Supports lat longitudinal & transverse arches
Nerve Superficial peroneal N (L5,S1)

PERONEUS TERTIUS
Arises Third quarter of ant shaft of fibula
Inserts Dorsal shaft & base of 5th MT
Action Extends & everts foot
Nerve Deep peroneal N (L5,S1)

PIRIFORMIS
Arises 2, 3, 4 costotransverse bars of ant sacrum between sacral foramina
Inserts Ant part of med aspect of greater trochanter of femur
Action Lat rotates & stabilises hip
Nerve Ant primary rami of S1,2
Notes Passes lat through greater sciatic foramen

PLANTARIS
Arises Lat supracondylar ridge of femur above lat head of gastrocnemius
Inserts Tendo calcaneus (med side, deep to gastrocnemius tendon)
Action Plantar flexes foot & flexes knee
Nerve Tibial N (S1,2)

PLATYSMA
Arises Skin over lower neck & upper lat chest
Inserts Inf border of mandible & skin over lower face & angle of mouth

8

Action Depresses & wrinkles skin of lower face & mouth. Aids forced depression of mandible

Nerve Cervical br of facial N (VII)

POPLITEUS

Arises Post shaft of tibia above soleal line & below tibial condyles

Inserts A facet on lat surface of lat condyle of femur postero-inferior to epicondyle. Tendon passes into capsule of knee and a few fibres attach to lat meniscus

Action Unlocks extended knee by lat rotation of femur on tibia. Pulls back lat meniscus

Nerve Tibial N (L4,5,S1)

Notes Popliteus bursa lies deep to tendon

POSTERIOR CRICOARYTENOID

Arises Post aspect of cricoid cartilage

Inserts Muscular process of arytenoid cartilage

Action Abducts & lat rotates arytenoid cartilage (opens rima glottidis)

Nerve Recurrent laryngeal br of vagus N (X)

PROCERUS

Arises Nasal bone & cartilages

Inserts Skin of med forehead

Action Wrinkles & 'frowns' forehead

Nerve Temporal br of facial N (VII)

PRONATOR QUADRATUS

Arises Lower quarter of anteromedial shaft of ulna

Inserts Lower quarter of anterolateral shaft of radius & some interosseous membrane

Action Pronates forearm & maintains ulna & radius opposed

Nerve Ant interosseous N (C8,T1)

PRONATOR TERES

Arises Humeral head: med epicondyle, med supracondylar ridge & med intermuscular septum. Ulnar head: med border of coronoid process

Inserts Just post to most prominent part of lat convexity of radius

Action Pronates forearm & flexes elbow

Nerve Median N (C6,7) (from lat & med cords)

Notes Median N passes between its two heads

PSOAS MAJOR

Arises Transverse processes of L1–5, bodies of T12–L5 & intervertebral discs below bodies of T12–L4

Inserts Middle surface of lesser trochanter of femur

Action Flexes hip

Nerve Ant primary rami of L1,2

PSOAS MINOR

Arises Bodies of T12 & L1 & intervening intervertebral disc

Inserts Pectineal line of pubis & fascia over iliopsoas

Action Weak flexor of trunk

Nerve Ant primary rami of L1

PYRAMIDALIS

Arises Public crest ant to origin of rectus abdominis

Inserts Lower linea alba

Action Reinforces lower rectus sheath

Nerve Subcostal N (T12)

QUADRATUS FEMORIS

Arises Lat border of ischial tuberosity

Inserts Quadrate tubercle of femur & a vertical line below this to the level of lesser trochanter

Action Lat rotates & stabilises hip

Nerve N to quadratus femoris (L4,5,S1)

QUADRATUS LUMBORUM

Arises Inf border of 12th rib

Inserts Apices of transverse processes of L1–4, iliolumbar lig & post third of iliac crest

8

Action Fixes 12th rib during respiration &
lat flexes trunk
Nerve Ant primary rami (T12–L3)

RECTUS ABDOMINIS
Arises Pubic crest & pubic symphysis
Inserts 5, 6, 7 costal cartilages, med inf
costal margin & post aspect of xiphoid
Action Flexes trunk, aids forced expiration
& raises intra-abdominal pressure
Nerve Ant primary rami (T7–12)

RECTUS CAPITIS ANTERIOR
Arises Lat mass of atlas (C1)
Inserts Basilar occipital bone ant to
occipital condyle
Action Flexes atlanto-occipital jnt
Nerve Ant primary rami of C1

RECTUS CAPITIS LATERALIS
Arises Lat mass of atlas (C1)
Inserts Jugular process of occipital bone
Action Lat flexes atlanto-occipital jnt
Nerve Ant primary rami of C1

RECTUS CAPITIS POSTERIOR MAJOR
Arises Spinous process of axis (C2)
Inserts Lat half of inf nuchal line
Action Extends & rotates atlanto-occipital
jnt
Nerve Suboccipital N (post primary ramus
C1)

RECTUS CAPITIS POSTERIOR MINOR
Arises Post process of atlas (C1)
Inserts Med half of inf nuchal line
Action Extends atlanto-occipital jnt
Nerve Suboccipital N (post primary ramus
C1)

RECTUS FEMORIS (QUADRICEPS FEMORIS I)
Arises Straight head: ant inf iliac spine.
Reflected head: ilium above acetabulum

Inserts Quadriceps tendon to patella, via
ligamentum patellae into tubercle of tibia
Action Extends leg at knee. Flexes thigh at
hip
Nerve Post div of femoral N (L2,3,4)

RHOMBOID MAJOR
Arises Spines of T2–T5 & supraspinous ligs
Inserts Lower half of posteromedial border
of scapula, from angle to upper part of
triangular area at base of scapular spine
Action Retracts scapula. Rotates scapula to
rest position
Nerve Dorsal scapular N (C5) (from root)

RHOMBOID MINOR
Arises Lower ligamentum nuchae, spines of
C7 & T1
Inserts Small area of posteromedial border
of scapula at level of spine, below levator
scapulae
Action Retracts scapula. Rotates scapula to
rest position
Nerve Dorsal scapular N (C5) (from root)

RISORIUS
Arises Deep fascia of face & parotid
Inserts Modiolus & skin at angle of mouth
Action Retracts angle of mouth
Nerve Buccal br of facial N (VII)

SALPINGOPHARYNGEUS
Arises Inf cartilage & mucosa of
pharyngeal orifice of auditory tube
Inserts Upper border of thyroid cartilage &
inf constrictor muscle fibres
Action Elevates pharynx & larynx & aids
swallowing. Opens auditory tube during
swallowing
Nerve Pharyngeal plexus (IX, X,
sympathetic) via pharyngeal br of vagus
N (X) with its motor fibres from cranial
accessory N (XI)

SARTORIUS
Arises Immediately below ant sup iliac spine

8

Inserts Upper med surface of shaft of tibia

Action Flexes, abducts, lat rotates thigh at hip. Flexes, med rotates leg at knee

Nerve Ant div of femoral N (L2,3)

SCALENUS ANTERIOR

Arises Ant tubercles of transverse processes of C3–6

Inserts Scalene tubercle on sup aspect of 1st rib

Action Accessory to inspiration. Lat flexion of neck when 1st rib fixed

Nerve Ant primary rami of C5,6

SCALENUS MEDIUS

Arises Post tubercles of transverse processes of C2–7

Inserts Sup aspect of 1st rib, ant to its tubercle

Action Accessory to inspiration

Nerve Ant primary rami of C3–8

SCALENUS MINIMUS

Arises Ant tubercle of transverse process of C7

Inserts Suprapleural membrane (Sibson's fascia)

Action Supports suprapleural membrane

Nerve Ant primary rami of C7

SCALENUS POSTERIOR

Arises Post tubercles of transverse processes C4–6

Inserts Posterolateral surface of 2nd rib

Action Accessory to inspiration

Nerve Ant primary rami of C6–8

SEMIMEMBRANOSUS

Arises Upper outer quadrant of post surface of ischial tuberosity

Inserts Med condyle of tibia below articular margin, fascia over popliteus & oblique popliteal lig

Action Flexes & med rotates knee. Extends hip

Nerve Tibial portion of sciatic N (L5,S1,2)

SEMITENDINOSUS

Arises Upper inner quadrant of post surface of ischial tuberosity

Inserts Upper med shaft of tibia behind gracilis

Action Flexes & med rotates knee. Extends hip

Nerve Tibial portion of sciatic N (L5,S1,2)

SERRATUS ANTERIOR

Arises Upper eight ribs & ant intercostal membranes from midclavicular line. Lower four interdigitating with external oblique

Inserts Inner med border scapula. 1 & 2: upper angle; 3 & 4: length of costal surface; 5–8: inf angle

Action Lat rotates & protracts scapula

Nerve Long thoracic N of Bell (C5,6,7) (from roots) slips from ribs 1 & 2: C5; 3 & 4: C6; 5–8: C7

SERRATUS POSTERIOR INFERIOR

Arises Spinous processes & supraspinous ligs of T11–L2

Inserts Post aspect of ribs 9–12

Action Assists forced expiration

Nerve Ant primary rami (T9–12)

SERRATUS POSTERIOR SUPERIOR

Arises Spinous processes & supraspinous lig of C7–T2

Inserts Post aspect of ribs 2–5

Action Assists forced inspiration

Nerve Ant primary rami (T2–5)

SOLEUS

Arises Soleal line & middle third of post border of tibia & upper quarter of post shaft of fibula including neck

Inserts Tendo calcaneus to middle of three facets on post surface of calcaneus

Action Plantar flexes foot (aids venous return)

Nerve Tibial N (S1,2)

Notes Main propulsive force for walking & running

8

SPHINCTER ANI (external)
Arises Circular anatomical sphincter
Inserts Deep, superficial & subcutaneous
   portions
Action Maintains continence of faeces
Nerve Inf rectal br of pudendal N (S2,3,4)

SPHINCTER URETHRAE
Arises Circular anatomical sphincter
Inserts Fuses with deep transverse perinei
Action Maintains continence of urine
Nerve Perineal br of pudendal N (S2,3,4)

SPLENIUS CAPITIS
Arises Lower lig nuchae, spinous processes
   & supraspinous ligs C7–T3
Inserts Lat occiput between sup & inf
   nuchal lines
Action Extends & rotates cervical spine
Nerve Post primary rami of C3,4

SPLENIUS CERVICIS
Arises Spinous processes & supraspinous
   ligs of T3–6
Inserts Post tubercles of transverse
   processes of C1–3
Action Extends & rotates cervical spine
Nerve Post primary rami of C5,6

STAPEDIUS
Arises The pyramid (post wall of middle ear)
Inserts Neck of stapes
Action Protects & critically damps
   ossicular chain
Nerve Facial N (VII), in middle ear

STERNOCLEIDOMASTOID
Arises Ant & sup manubrium &
   superomedial third of clavicle
Inserts Lat aspect of mastoid process & ant
   half of sup nuchal line
Action Acting alone it laterally flexes
   cervical spine & rotates head on neck to
   bring ipsilateral ear to ipsilateral shoulder.
   Acting together they protrude head & if
   head is fixed, aid respiration

Nerve Spinal root of accessory N (XI)
   (lat roots C1–5)
Notes Effectively four separate muscles

STERNOHYOID
Arises Sup lat post aspect of manubrium
Inserts Inf border of body of hyoid bone
Action Depresses hyoid bone & hence
   larynx
Nerve Ansa cervicalis N (C1,2,3)

STERNOTHYROID
Arises Med post aspect of manubrium
Inserts Oblique line of lamina of thyroid
   cartilage
Action Depresses larynx
Nerve Ansa cervicalis N (C1,2,3)

STYLOGLOSSUS
Arises Ant surface & apex of styloid
   process & upper quarter of stylohyoid lig
Inserts Superolateral sides of tongue
Action Retracts & elevates tongue, aids
   initiation of swallowing
Nerve Hypoglossal N (XII)

STYLOHYOID
Arises Base of styloid process
Inserts Base of greater cornu of hyoid bone
Action Elevates & retracts hyoid bone.
   Aids swallowing & elevates larynx
Nerve Facial N (VII) before it enters
   parotid gland

STYLOPHARYNGEUS
Arises Med aspect of styloid process
Inserts Posterolateral border of thyroid
   cartilage
Action Elevates larynx & pharynx. Aids
   swallowing
Nerve Muscular br of glossopharyngeal N
   (IX)

SUBCLAVIUS
Arises Costochondral junction of 1st rib

8

Inserts Subclavian groove on inf surface of middle third of clavicle

Action Depresses clavicle & steadies it during shoulder movements

Nerve N to subclavius (C5,6, upper trunk)

SUBCOSTALIS

Arises Int post aspects of lower six ribs

Inserts Int aspects of ribs two to three levels below

Action Depresses lower ribs

Nerve Muscular collateral brs of intercostal Ns

Notes Subcostalis is one of three muscles that make up inner layer of thoracic wall muscles. Others are innermost intercostals (lat) & transversus thoracis (ant)

SUBSCAPULARIS

Arises Med two-thirds of subscapular fossa

Inserts Lesser tuberosity of humerus, upper med lip of bicipital groove, capsule of shoulder jnt

Action Med rotates arm & stabilises shoulder jnt

Nerve Upper & lower subscapular Ns (C5,6) (from post cord)

Notes Subscapular bursa beneath tendon, usually connected with jnt. Tendon forms part of rotator cuff

SUPERFICIAL TRANSVERSE PERINEI

Arises Body of ischium

Inserts Perineal body

Action Fixes perineal body

Nerve Perineal br of pudendal N (S2,3,4)

SUPERIOR OBLIQUE (see also obliquus capitis superior)

Arises Body of sphenoid superomedial to tendinous ring

Inserts Post/sup quadrant of sclera behind equator of eyeball on lat side

Action Depresses eye in adduction. Intorts eye in abduction

Nerve Trochlear N (IV)

Notes Passes around trochlear sling on frontal bone

SUPERIOR RECTUS

Arises Sup tendinous ring within orbit

Inserts Sup sclera ant to equator of eyeball

Action Elevates eye. Intorts eye in adduction

Nerve Sup div of oculomotor N (III)

SUPINATOR

Arises Deep part (horizontal): supinator crest & fossa of ulna. Superficial part (downwards): lat epicondyle & lat lig of elbow & annular lig

Inserts Neck & shaft of radius, between ant & post oblique lines

Action Supinates forearm. Only acts alone when elbow extended

Nerve Post interosseous N (C6,7)

Notes Post interosseous N passes between its two heads

SUPRASPINATUS

Arises Med three-quarters of supraspinous fossa of scapula, upper surface of spine (bipennate)

Inserts Sup facet on greater tuberosity of humerus & capsule of shoulder jnt

Action Abducts arm & stabilises shoulder jnt

Nerve Suprascapular N (C5,6) (from upper trunk)

Notes Subacromial bursa lies above its tendon. Tendon forms part of rotator cuff

TEMPORALIS

Arises Temporal fossa between inf temporal line & infratemporal crest

Inserts Med & ant aspects of coronoid process of mandible

Action Elevates mandible & post fibres retract it

Nerve Deep temporal brs from ant div of mandibular N (Vc)

8

TEMPOROPARIETALIS
Arises Aponeurosis above ear
Inserts Galeal aponeurosis
Action Fixes galeal aponeurosis
Nerve Temporal br of facial N (VII)

TENSOR FASCIAE LATAE
Arises Outer surface of ant iliac crest between tubercle of the iliac crest & ant sup iliac spine
Inserts Iliotibial tract (ant surface of lat condyle of tibia)
Action Maintains knee extended (assists gluteus maximus) & abducts hip
Nerve Sup gluteal N (L4,5,S1)

TENSOR TYMPANI
Arises Cartilaginous & bony margins of auditory tube
Inserts Handle of malleus (via processus trochleariformis)
Action Protects & critically damps ossicular chain
Nerve Off N to med pterygoid (main trunk of mandibular N (Vc))

TENSOR VELI PALATINI
Arises Scaphoid fossa, med aspect of spine of sphenoid bone & lat cartilage of auditory tube
Inserts Palatine aponeurosis (via pulley of pterygoid hamulus)
Action Tenses soft palate prior to elevation. Opens auditory tube on swallowing
Nerve Off N to med pterygoid (main trunk of mandibular N (Vc))

TERES MAJOR
Arises Oval area (lower third) of lat side of inf angle of scapula below teres minor
Inserts Med lip of bicipital groove of humerus
Action Med rotates & adducts arm. Stabilises shoulder jnt
Nerve Lower subscapular N (C5,6,7) (from post cord)
Notes Functionally part of subscapularis

TERES MINOR
Arises Middle third lat border of scapula above teres major
Inserts Inf facet of greater tuberosity of humerus (below infraspinatus) & capsule of shoulder jnt
Action Lat rotates arm & stabilises shoulder jnt
Nerve Axillary N (C5,6) (from post cord)
Notes Functionally part of infraspinatus. Tendon forms part of rotator cuff

THYRO-ARYTENOID & VOCALIS
Arises Lower post surface of angle between laminae of thyroid cartilage
Inserts Vocal process of arytenoid cartilage
Action Shortens & relaxes vocal cords by approximating arytenoid cartilage to thyroid cartilage
Nerve Recurrent laryngeal br of vagus N (X)
Notes Vocalis is that part of thyro-arytenoid that inserts into vocal cord itself

THYRO-EPIGLOTTICUS
Arises Lower post surface of thyroid cartilage
Inserts Lat border of epiglottis
Action Widens additus of larynx
Nerve Recurrent laryngeal br of vagus N (X)

THYROHYOID
Arises Oblique line on lamina of thyroid cartilage
Inserts Inf border of body of hyoid bone
Action Elevates larynx or depresses hyoid bone
Nerve C1 fibres carried by hypoglossal N (XII)

TIBIALIS ANTERIOR
Arises Upper half of lat shaft of tibia & interosseous membrane
Inserts Inferomedial aspect of med cuneiform & base of 1st MT

8

Action Extends & inverts foot at ankle. Holds up med longitudinal arch of foot
Nerve Deep peroneal N (L4,5)
Notes Inversion is at subtalar & mid tarsal joints

TIBIALIS POSTERIOR

Arises Upper half of post shaft of tibia & upper half of fibula between median crest & interosseous border, & interosseous membrane
Inserts Tuberosity of navicular bone & all tarsal bones (except talus) & bases of metatarsals 2–4
Action Plantar flexes & inverts foot. Supports med longitudinal arch of foot
Nerve Tibial N (L4,5)

TRANSVERSE ARYTENOID

Arises Post surface & muscular process of arytenoid cartilage
Inserts Corresponding surfaces of opposite cartilage
Action Adducts arytenoid cartilages (closes rima glottidis)
Nerve Recurrent laryngeal branch of vagus N (X)

TRANSVERSOSPINALIS— MULTIFIDUS

Arises Laminae of vertebra from sacrum to C2
Inserts Spinous processes two to three levels above
Action Extends spine
Nerve Post primary rami

TRANSVERSOSPINALIS— ROTATORES

Arises Transverse processes
Inserts Spinous processes one above
Action Rotates spine
Nerve Post primary rami
Notes Two types—thoracis & cervicis et lumborum

TRANSVERSOSPINALIS— SEMISPINALIS

Arises Transverse processes
Inserts Spinous processes six levels above
Action Extends & lat flexes spine
Nerve Post primary rami
Notes Three types—thoracis, cervicis & capitis

TRANSVERSUS ABDOMINIS

Arises Costal margin (ribs & costal cartilages), lumbar fascia, ant two-thirds of iliac crest & lat half of inguinal lig
Inserts Aponeurosis of post & ant rectus sheath & conjoint tendon to pubic crest & pectineal line
Action Supports abdominal wall, aids forced expiration & raising intra-abdominal pressure. Conjoint tendon supports post wall of inguinal canal
Nerve Ant primary rami (T7–12). Conjoint tendon: ilio-inguinal N (L1)

TRANSVERSUS THORACIS (STERNOCOSTALIS)

Arises Lower third of inner aspect of sternum & lower three costosternal junctions
Inserts Second to sixth costal cartilages
Action Depresses upper ribs
Nerve Muscular collateral brs of intercostal Ns
Notes Transversus thoracis is one of three muscles that make up inner layer of thoracic wall muscles. Others are innermost intercostals (lat) & subcostals (post)

TRAPEZIUS

Arises Med third sup nuchal line, lig nuchae, spinous processes & supraspinous ligs to T12
Inserts Upper fibres to lat third of post border of clavicle; med acromion & lat spine of scapula. Lower fibres to med end of spine of scapula as far as deltoid tubercle
Action Elevates & retracts scapula. Rotates it during abduction of arm. If scapula is fixed, extends & lat flexes neck

8

Nerve Spinal root of accessory N (XI) (lat roots, C1–5) (spinal nerves C3 & C4 for proprioception)

TRICEPS

Arises Long head: infraglenoid tubercle of scapula. Lat head: upper half post humerus (linear origin). Med head: lower half post humerus inferomedial to spiral groove & both intermuscular septa

Inserts Post part of upper surface of olecranon process of ulna & post capsule

Action Extends elbow. Long head stabilises shoulder jnt. Med head retracts capsule of elbow jnt on extension

Nerve Radial N (C6,7,8) (from post cord), four brs

VASTUS INTERMEDIUS (QUADRICEPS FEMORIS 2)

Arises Ant & lat shaft of femur to one hand's breadth above condyles

Inserts Quadriceps tendon to patella, via ligamentum patellae into tubercle of tibia

Action Extends knee

Nerve Post div of femoral N (L2,3,4)

VASTUS LATERALIS (QUADRICEPS FEMORIS 3)

Arises Upper intertrochanteric line, base of greater trochanter, lat linea aspera, lat

supracondylar ridge & lat intermuscular septum

Inserts Lat quadriceps tendon to patella, via ligamentum patellae into tubercle of tibia

Action Extends knee

Nerve Post div of femoral N (L2,3,4)

VASTUS MEDIALIS (QUADRICEPS FEMORIS 4)

Arises Lower intertrochanteric line, spiral line, med linea aspera & med intermuscular septum

Inserts Med quadriceps tendon to patella & directly into med patella, via ligamentum patellae into tubercle of tibia

Action Extends knee. Stabilises patella

Nerve Post div of femoral N (L2,3,4)

ZYGOMATICUS MAJOR

Arises Ant surface of zygomatic bone

Inserts Modiolus at angle of mouth

Action Elevates & draws angle of mouth laterally

Nerve Buccal br of facial N (VII)

ZYGOMATICUS MINOR

Arises Lat infra-orbital margin

Inserts Skin & muscle of upper lip

Action Elevates & everts upper lip

Nerve Buccal br of facial N (VII)

8

Aide memoir for nerve supply of groups of muscles in head and neck

All muscles of:	Supplied by:	Except:	Which is supplied by:
Pharynx	Pharyngeal plexus (IX, X, sympathetic)	Stylopharyngeus	Glossopharyngeal (IX)
Palate	Pharyngeal plexus (IX, X, sympathetic)	Tensor palati	Off N to med pterygoid (Vc)
Tongue	Hypoglossal (XII)	Palatoglossus	Pharyngeal plexus (IX, X, sympathetic)
Mastication	Mandibular (Vc)	Buccinator	Facial (VII)
Larynx	Recurrent laryngeal (X)	Cricothyroid	Ext br of superior laryngeal (X)
Facial expression & buccinator	Facial (VII)		

9: JOINTS

Classification of joints

Fibrous Fibrous tissue between bones
Primary cartilaginous Hyaline cartilage between bones
Secondary cartilaginous As for primary but fibrocartilage between the layers of hyaline cartilage (symphysis)
Synovial Joint cavity with synovial fluid. Hyaline cartilage on surface of bones. Articular disc can be present
Atypical synovial Joint cavity with synovial fluid. Fibrocartilage on surface of bones. Articular disc can be present

Types of synovial joint

Plane Sliding only
Hinge (ginglymus) One plane of movement
Modified hinge (bicondylar) One plane of movement + rotation
Condyloid (ellipsoid) Two planes of movement (circumduction)
Saddle condyloid (sella) Two planes of movement + controlled rotation
Pivot (trochoid) Rotation only. One plane of movement
Ball and socket (spheroidal) Multi-axial. Three planes of movement

Joints with interarticular fibrocartilaginous discs

Acromioclavicular (usually incomplete)
Femorotibial (knee) (incomplete—menisci)
Radiocarpal (wrist)
Sternoclavicular
Temporomandibular

Joints with double cavities separated by intra-articular ligaments—not fibrocartilaginous discs

Costovertebral (ribs 2–10)
Sternochondral (2nd rib)

Joints classified by type

Fibrous joints
Arytenocorniculate (can be synovial)
Costotransverse (ribs 11 and 12)
Cuboideonavicular (can be synovial)
Gomphosis (teeth)
Radio-ulnar (interosseous membrane)
Skull sutures
Tibiofibular (inferior)
Tibiofibular (interosseous membrane)

Primary cartilaginous joints
Costochondral
Sternochondral (1st rib)
Spheno-occipital

Secondary cartilaginous joints
Intervertebral
Manubriosternal
Sacrococcygeal
Symphysis pubis
Xiphisternal

Atypical synovial joints
Acromioclavicular
Sternochondral (ribs 2–7)
Sternoclavicular
Temporomandibular

Typical synovial
Acetabulofemoral (hip)
Atlanto-axial (dens & facets)
Atlanto-occipital
Calcaneocuboid
Carpometacarpal
Costotransverse (ribs 1–10)

9

Costovertebral
Crico-arytenoid
Crico-thyroid
Cuneocuboid
Cuneonavicular
Femorotibial (knee)
Glenohumeral (shoulder)
Humeroradial (elbow)
Humero-ulnar (elbow)
Intercarpal
Interchondral (cartilages 6–10)
Intercuneiform
Intermetacarpal
Intermetatarsal
Interphalangeal
Metacarpophalangeal
Metatarsophalangeal
Pisotriquetral
Radiocarpal (wrist)
Radio-ulnar (superior & inferior)
Talocalcaneal
Talocalcaneonavicular
Tarsometatarsal
Tibiofibular (superior)
Tibiotalal (ankle)
Zygapophyseal (intervertebral facet)

Unclassified

Intervertebral joints of Luschka

Named joints

Acetabulofemoral (hip)   180
Acromioclavicular   180
Ankle (see tibiotalal)
Arytenocorniculate (larynx)   180
Atlanto-axial—lateral   180
Atlanto-axial—median   180
Atlanto-occipital   180
Calcaneocuboid (midtarsal)   180
Carpometacarpal—fingers 2–5 (including
    intermetacarpal)   180
Carpometacarpal—thumb   180
Costochondral   180
Costotransverse—ribs 1–10   180
Costotransverse—ribs 11, 12   180
Costovertebral   180
Crico-arytenoid (larynx)   180
Cricothyroid (larynx)   181
Cuboideonavicular (see intertarsal)

Cuneocuboid (see intertarsal)
Cuneonavicular (see intertarsal)
Elbow (see humero-ulnar, humeroradial &
    superior radio-ulnar)   181
Facet (vertebral articulations) (see
    zygapophyseal)
Femorotibial (knee)   181
Glenohumeral (shoulder)   181
Gomphosis (dento-alveolar)   181
Hip (see acetabulofemoral)
Humeroradial (elbow)   181
Humero-ulnar (elbow)   181
Intercarpal (midcarpal) (see also
    pisotriquetral)
Interchondral   181
Intercuneiform (see intertarsal)
Intermetacarpal (see carpometacarpal—
    fingers 2–5)
Intermetatarsal   181
Interphalangeal (fingers & toes)   181
Intertarsal—cuboideonavicular   181
Intertarsal—cuneocuboid   181
Intertarsal—cuneonavicular   182
Intertarsal—intercuneiform   182
Intervertebral   182
Intervertebral facets
    (see zygapophyseal)
Intervertebral joints of Luschka
    (neurocentral or uncovertebral)   182
Knee (see femorotibial)
Manubriosternal   182
Metacarpophalangeal   182
Metatarsophalangeal   182
Midcarpal (see intercarpal)
Midtarsal (see calcaneocuboid &
    talonavicular part of
    talocalcaneonavicular)
Pelvic (see sacro-iliac & symphysis
    pubis)
Pisotriquetral   182
Radiocarpal (wrist)   182
Radio-ulnar—inferior   182
Radio-ulnar—interosseous membrane &
    oblique cord   182
Radio-ulnar—superior   182
Sacrococcygeal   182
Sacro-iliac   182
Shoulder (see glenohumeral)
Skull sutures   183
Spheno-occipital   183
Sternochondral (sternocostal)   183

9

All joints are paired except the following
which are single midline joints:
Median atlanto-axial
Intervertebral
Manubriosternal
Spheno-occipital
Symphysis pubis
Xiphisternal

9

ACETABULOFEMORAL (hip)
Classification Synovial
Type Ball & socket
Articulation Acetabulum with femur

ACROMIOCLAVICULAR
Classification Atypical synovial
Type Plane
Articulation Acromion with clavicle
Notes Often an articular disc in upper part
  of jnt, usually incomplete

ANKLE (see tibiotalal)

ARYTENOCORNICULATE (larynx)
Classification Fibrous or synovial
Articulation Arytenoid cartilage with
  corniculate cartilage

ATLANTO-AXIAL—LATERAL
Classification Synovial
Type Plane
Articulation Articular facets of atlas with
  axis

ATLANTO-AXIAL—MEDIAN
Classification Synovial
Type Pivot
Articulation Dens of axis with atlas
Notes Second cavity (bursa) posteriorly

ATLANTO-OCCIPITAL
Classification Synovial
Type Condyloid
Articulation Atlas with occipital bone

CALCANEOCUBOID (midtarsal)
Classification Synovial
Type Saddle condyloid
Articulation Calcaneus with cuboid
Notes This is one part of midtarsal jnt.
  Other is talonavicular part of
  talocalcaneonavicular

CARPOMETACARPAL—FINGERS 2–5
(including intermetacarpal)
Classification Synovial
Type Plane
Articulation Carpal bones with MCs &
  between MCs
Notes Usually continuous cavity between
  CMC, intermetacarpal & intercarpal jnts

CARPOMETACARPAL—THUMB
Classification Synovial
Type Saddle condyloid
Articulation Trapezium with 1st MC
Notes Joint is separate from others in hand

COSTOCHONDRAL
Classification Primary cartilaginous
Articulation Bony rib with costal cartilage

COSTOTRANSVERSE—RIBS 1–10
Classification Synovial
Type Plane
Articulation Med facet of tubercle of rib
  with transverse process of own vertebra

COSTOTRANSVERSE—RIBS 11, 12
Classification Fibrous (ligamentous)
Articulation Tubercle of rib with
  transverse process of own vertebra

COSTOVERTEBRAL
Classification Synovial
Type Plane
Articulation Head of rib with vertebral
  body
Notes 1st rib articulates with T1 vertebra
  only (single cavity jnt). Ribs 2–10 with
  own vertebra & one above (double cavity
  jnts separated by intra-articular lig). Ribs
  11 & 12 with own vertebra only (single
  cavity jnts)

CRICO-ARYTENOID (larynx)
Classification Synovial
Type Features of ball & socket

9

Articulation Cricoid cartilage with arytenoid cartilage

CRICOTHYROID (larynx)
Classification Synovial
Type Plane (rotational). Two together give hinge movement
Articulation Facet on side of cricoid cartilage with inf horn of thyroid cartilage

ELBOW (see humeroradial & humero-ulnar)

FEMOROTIBIAL (knee)
Classification Synovial
Type Modified hinge
Articulation Femur with tibia
Notes Menisci are incomplete discs of fibrocartilage

GLENOHUMERAL (shoulder)
Classification Synovial
Type Ball & socket
Articulation Glenoid fossa of scapula with humerus

GOMPHOSIS (dento-alveolar)
Classification Fibrous
Articulation Tooth with bone of jaw

HIP (see acetabulofemoral)

HUMERORADIAL (elbow)
Classification Synovial
Type Hinge
Articulation Capitulum of humerus with radial head
Notes Jnt cavity is shared with humero-ulnar & sup radio-ulnar jnts

HUMERO-ULNAR (elbow)
Classification Synovial
Type Hinge

Articulation Trochlea of humerus with ulnar trochlear notch
Notes Jnt cavity is shared with humeroradial & sup radio-ulnar jnts

INTERCARPAL (MIDCARPAL)
(see also pisotriquetral)
Classification Synovial
Type Plane individually but together give effective mixture of condyloid, saddle condyloid & ball & socket
Articulation Between scaphoid, lunate, triquetral, hamate, capitate, trapezoid & trapezium
Notes Single cavity between the seven bones usually communicating also with CMC & intercarpal jnts of fingers 2–5

INTERCHONDRAL
Classification Synovial
Type Plane
Articulation Between costal cartilages 6/7, 7/8, 8/9, 9/10

INTERMETATARSAL
Classification Synovial
Type Plane
Articulation Between MTs

INTERPHALANGEAL (fingers & toes)
Classification Synovial
Type Hinge
Articulation Between phalanges

INTERTARSAL—CUBOIDEONAVICULAR
Classification Fibrous (can be synovial)
Articulation Cuboid with navicular

INTERTARSAL—CUNEOCUBOID
Classification Synovial
Type Plane
Articulation Lat cuneiform with cuboid
Notes Cuneocuboid shares cavity with cuneonavicular & intercuneiform jnts

9

INTERTARSAL—CUNEONAVICULAR
Classification Synovial
Type Plane
Articulation Cuneiforms with navicular
Notes Cuneonavicular shares cavity with cuneocuboid and intercuneiform jnts

INTERTARSAL—INTERCUNEIFORM
Classification Synovial
Type Plane
Articulation Between cuneiforms
Notes Intercuneiform jnts share cavity with cuneonavicular & cuneocuboid jnts

INTERVERTEBRAL
Classification Secondary cartilaginous
Articulation Between vertebral bodies

INTERVERTEBRAL JOINTS OF LUSCHKA (neurocentral or uncovertebral)
Classification Unclassified
Type Unclassified
Articulation Lateral lip of upper surface of C3–7 & T1 vertebrae with adjacent vertebral body above
Notes Often small cavity which is degenerative (not synovial)

KNEE (see femorotibial)

MANUBRIOSTERNAL
Classification Secondary cartilaginous
Articulation Manubrium with sternum
Notes May cavitate to give appearance of synovial jnt

METACARPOPHALANGEAL
Classification Synovial
Type Condyloid
Articulation MCs with phalanges

METATARSOPHALANGEAL
Classification Synovial
Type Condyloid
Articulation MTs with phalanges

MIDTARSAL (see both talonavicular part of talocalcaneonavicular and calcaneocuboid)

PISOTRIQUETRAL
Classification Synovial
Type Plane
Articulation Pisiform with triquetral

RADIOCARPAL (wrist)
Classification Synovial
Type Condyloid
Articulation Radius & triangular fibrocartilaginous articular disc with scaphoid, lunate & triquetral

RADIO-ULNAR—INFERIOR
Classification Synovial
Type Pivot
Articulation Radius with ulna
Notes Cavity separated from cavity of wrist by triangular fibrocartilaginous disc

RADIO-ULNAR—INTEROSSEOUS MEMBRANE & OBLIQUE CORD
Classification Fibrous
Articulation Radius with ulna

RADIO-ULNAR—SUPERIOR
Classification Synovial
Type Pivot
Articulation Radius with ulna
Notes Cavity is continuous with humero-ulnar & humeroradial jnts

SACROCOCCYGEAL
Classification Secondary cartilaginous
Articulation Sacrum with coccyx

SACRO-ILIAC
Classification Synovial

Type Plane
Articulation Sacrum with iliac bone

SHOULDER (see glenohumeral)

SKULL SUTURES
Classification Fibrous
Articulation Between diploae of skull

SPHENO-OCCIPITAL
Classification Primary cartilaginous
Articulation Sphenoid with basi-occiput

STERNOCHONDRAL (sternocostal)
Classification 1st: primary cartilaginous;
   2nd–7th: atypical synovial
Type 2nd–7th: plane
Articulation 1st rib with manubrium.
   3rd–7th ribs with sternum. 2nd with
   both
Notes 2nd jnt has two cavities separated by
   intra-articular lig

STERNOCLAVICULAR
(manubrioclavicular)
Classification Atypical synovial
Type Features of ball & socket
Articulation Clavicle with manubrium
Notes Separated into two cavities by
   fibrocartilaginous disc

SUBTALAR (see both talocalcanean &
talocalcaneal part of talocalcaneonavicular)

SYMPHYSIS PUBIS
Classification Secondary cartilaginous
Articulation Between pubic bones
Notes May cavitate

TALOCALCANEAN (subtalar)
Classification Synovial
Type Plane (effectively ball & socket)
Articulation Talus with calcaneus

Notes This is a posterior, separate jnt that is
   one-half of subtalar jnt

TALOCALCANEONAVICULAR
Classification Synovial
Type Features of ball & socket
Articulation Talus with calcaneus &
   navicular
Notes This is a two part jnt. Talocalcaneal
   part (two facets) is part of subtalar jnt,
   other being talocalcanean. Talonavicular
   part (one facet) is part of midtarsal jnt,
   other being calcaneocuboid.

TARSOMETATARSAL
Classification Synovial
Type Plane
Articulation Tarsal bones with MTs

TEMPOROMANDIBULAR
Classification Atypical synovial
Type Condyloid
Articulation Temporal bone with mandible
Notes Separated into two cavities by
   fibrocartilaginous disc

TIBIOFIBULAR—INFERIOR
Classification Fibrous
Articulation Tibia with fibula

**TIBIOFIBULAR—INTEROSSEOUS
MEMBRANE**
Classification Fibrous
Articulation Tibia with fibula

TIBIOFIBULAR—SUPERIOR
Classification Synovial
Type Plane
Articulation Tibia with fibula

TIBIOTALAL (ankle)
Classification Synovial
Type Hinge
Articulation Tibia with talus

9

WRIST (see radiocarpal & interarticular disc of inferior radio-ulnar)

XIPHISTERNAL
Classification Secondary cartilaginous
Articulation Xiphoid with sternum

ZYGAPOPHYSEAL (intervertebral facet)
Classification Synovial
Type Plane
Articulation Between intervertebral facets

10: OSSIFICATION TIMES

Ossification times

Bones (number if unpaired)	Forms in membrane (M) or cartilage (C)	Centres primary (P) or secondary (S)	Site	Centre appears at: Gestation (weeks/months)	After birth	Fused by
Mandible (1)	M	P	Near mental foramen (each side)	6 W		Symphysis menti 1–3 Y
Hyoid (1)	C	P	Greater cornu (each side)	8–9 M		
	C	S	Body (2 centres)	9 M		
	C	S	Lesser cornu (each side)		Puberty	
Occiput (1)	M	P	Squamous (each side)	8 W		
	C	P	Lateral (each side)	8 W		
	C	P	Basilar	8 W		
Sphenoid (1)	M+C	P	Approximately 14 centres	8 W–4 M		
Temporal	M	P	Squamous	8 W		
	M	P	Tympanic	3 M		
	C	P	Petromastoid (several centres)	5 M		
Parietal	M	P	Near tuberosity (2 centres)	7 W		
Frontal (2 → 1)	M	P	Near each tuberosity (2 centres, one each side)	8 W		Metopic suture 2 Y
Ethmoid (1)	C	P	Labyrinth (one each side)	5 M		
	C	P	Perpendicular plate/crista galli		1 Y	
Inf concha	M	P		5 M		
Lacrimal	M	P		4 M		
Nasal	M	P		3 M		
Vomer (1)	M	P	(2 centres)	8 W		
Maxilla	M	P	(3 centres)	6–8 W		
Palatine	M	P	Perpendicular plate	8 W		

				Appears	Fuses
Zygomatic		M	P	8 W	
Ear ossicles	Stapes	C	P	4 M	
	Malleus	C	P	4 M	
	Incus	C	P	4 M	
Scapula	Body	C	P	8 W	
	Coracoid process	C	S	1 Y	15 Y
	Subcoracoid	C	S	Puberty	20 Y
	Medial border	C	S	Puberty	20 Y
	Glenoid (lower rim)	C	S	Puberty	20 Y
	Acromion (2 centres)	C	S	Puberty	20 Y
	Inferior angle	C	S	Puberty	20 Y
Clavicle	Medial & lateral (2 centres)	M	P	5 W	
	Sternal end	M	S	Late teens	20 Y
Humerus (upper end is growing end)	Shaft	C	P	8 W	
	Head	C	S	6 M	Upper epiphysis 18–20 Y
	Greater tuberosity	C	S	2 Y	
	Lesser tuberosity	C	S	5 Y	
	Capitulum & lat ridge of trochlea	C	S	1 Y	
	Medial trochlea	C	S	10 Y	
	Medial epicondyle	C	S	5 Y	Lower epiphysis 14–16 Y
	Lateral epicondyle	C	S	12 Y	
Radius (lower end is growing end)	Shaft	C	P	8 W	
	Head	C	S	4 Y	14–17 Y
	Distal end	C	S	1 Y	17–19 Y
Ulna (lower end is growing end)	Shaft	C	P	8 W	
	Olecranon (2 centres)	C	S	9 Y	14–16 Y
	Distal end	C	S	5 Y	17–18 Y
Carpus	Capitate	C	P	2 M	
	Hamate	C	P	3 M	
	Triquetral	C	P	3 Y	
	Lunate	C	P	4 Y	

continued on p. 188

10

Ossification times *continued*

Bones (number if unpaired)	Forms in membrane (M) or cartilage (C)	Centres primary (P) or secondary (S)	Site	Centre appears at: Gestation (weeks/months)	After birth	Fused by
	C	P	Scaphoid		4–5 Y	
	C	P	Trapezium		4–5 Y	
	C	P	Trapezoid		4–5 Y	
	C	P	Pisiform		9–12 Y	
Metacarpal (1st)	C	P	Shaft	9 W		
	C	S	Base		3 Y	15–17 Y
Metacarpals (2nd–5th)	C	P	Shaft	9 W		
	C	S	Head		2 Y	15–19 Y
Phalanges (hand)	C	P	Shaft	8–12 W		
	C	S	Base		2–4 Y	15–18 Y
Innominate	C	P	Pubis (superior ramus)	4 M		7–8 Y
	C	P	Ischium (body)	4 M		7–8 Y
	C	P	Ilium (above greater sciatic notch)	2 M		7–8 Y
	C	S	Iliac crest (2 centres)		Puberty	15–25 Y
	C	S	Acetabulum (2 centres)		Puberty	15–25 Y
	C	S	Anterior superior iliac spine		Puberty	15–25 Y
	C	S	Ischial tuberosity		Puberty	15–25 Y
	C	S	Pubic symphysis		Puberty	15–25 Y
Femur (lower end is growing end)	C	P	Shaft	7 W		
	C	S	Greater trochanter		4 Y	
	C	S	Lesser trochanter		12 Y	
	C	S	Head		6 M	
	C	S	Distal end	9 M		14–17 Y
						16–18 Y
Patella	C	P	(Several centres)		3–6 Y	Puberty
	C	S	Superolaterally		6 Y	Puberty

10

			Appears	Fuses
Tibia (upper end is growing end)				
Shaft	P	C	7 W	16–18 Y
Plateau	S	C	9 M	15–17 Y
Distal end	S	C	1 Y	13–14 Y
Tuberosity	S	C	12 Y	
Fibula (upper end is growing end)				
Shaft	P	C	8 W	15–17 Y
Distal end	S	C	1 Y	17–19 Y
Head	S	C	3–4 Y	
Talus	P	C	6 M	
Calcaneus	P	C	3 M	
	S	C	6–8 Y	14–16 Y
Navicular	P	C	3 Y	
Cuneiform lateral	P	C	1 Y	
Cuneiform medial (May have 2 centres)	P	C	2 Y	
Cuneiform intermediate	P	C	3 Y	
Cuboid	P	C	9 M	
Metatarsal (1st)				
Shaft	P	C	9 W	17–20 Y
Base	S	C	3 Y	17–20 Y
Metatarsals (2nd–5th)				
Shaft	P	C	9 W	17–20 Y
Head	S	C	3–4 Y	17–20 Y
Phalanges (foot)				
Shaft	P	C	9–15 W	18 Y
Base	S	C	2–8 Y	18 Y

continued on p. 190

Closure of skull sutures

Ant fontinelle: closes 18 M; post fontinelle: closes 6 M–1 Y

Notes: (1) All bones are paired unless otherwise stated. (2) Single centre of ossification unless specified otherwise. (3) Variability of ossification usually a sex difference, females appearing and uniting earlier. (4) Fusion times for epiphyses are given if clinically relevant

10

Ossification times *continued*—eruption of teeth

Eruption of teeth

	Incisor		Canine	Premolar	Molar
	(upper)	(lower)			
First dentition (months)	7, 8	6, 9	18		12, 24
Second dentition* (years)	7, 8	7, 8	11	9, 10	6, 12, 18

* Lower teeth erupt slightly earlier.

10

11: FORAMINA—SKULL AND SPINE

Notes: (1) Most smaller emissary veins and meningeal arterial supplies have been omitted. (2) All structures are paired unless otherwise indicated.

11

AQUEDUCT OF THE VESTIBULE

Site In post aspect of petrous temporal bone in post cranial fossa, 1 cm post to int acoustic meatus

Contains Endolymphatic duct & sac, small art & V

CAROTID CANAL

Site In inf surface of petrous temporal bone in middle cranial fossa

Contains Int carotid art enters with sympathetic plexus on it. Int carotid venous plexus connecting cavernous sinus & int jugular vein

CONDYLAR CANAL

Site In lower sigmoid groove in occipital bone in post cranial fossa. Exits at condylar fossa behind condyle (not always present)

Contains Emissary V connecting sigmoid sinus & occipital Vs. Meningeal br of occipital art

CRIBRIFORM FORAMINA

Site In cribriform plate of ethmoid bone in ant cranial fossa

Contains Olfactory filaments & ant ethmoidal N & vessels

FACIAL CANAL

Site In petrous temporal bone leading from int acoustic meatus to stylomastoid foramen

Contains Facial N (VII)

FORAMEN CAECUM (unpaired)

Site Between frontal crest of frontal bone & crista galli of ethmoid bone in ant cranial fossa

Contains Emissary Vs connecting nose & sup sagittal sinus

FORAMEN LACERUM

Site Between sphenoid, apex of petrous temporal & basilar occipital bones in middle cranial fossa

Contains Int carotid art enters behind & exits above. Greater petrosal N enters behind/above & leaves ant as N of the pterygoid canal

FORAMEN MAGNUM (unpaired)

Site In occipital bone in post cranial fossa

Contains Medulla oblongata, meninges, vertebral arts, ant & post spinal arts, spinal roots of accessory Ns (XI), sympathetic plexus on vertebral art, apical ligament of dens, tectorial membrane

FORAMEN OVALE

Site In greater wing of sphenoid bone in middle cranial fossa

Contains Mandibular N (Vc), lesser petrosal N, accessory meningeal art

FORAMEN ROTUNDUM

Site In greater wing of sphenoid bone in middle cranial fossa

Contains Maxillary N (Vb)

FORAMEN SPINOSUM

Site In greater wing of sphenoid bone in middle cranial fossa

Contains Middle meningeal vessels, meningeal br of mandibular N (Vc)

FORAMEN TRANSVERSARIUM

Site In pedicle of cervical vertebrae bordered by—lat: intertubercular lamella (costotransverse bar), med: body of vertebra

Contains Vertebral art & V in C1–6. Vein only in C7

GREATER PALATINE FORAMEN

Site Between maxilla & palatine bone at lat edge of hard palate

Contains Greater palatine N & vessels

HYPOGLOSSAL CANAL
Site In occipital bone above condyle in post cranial fossa
Contains Hypoglossal N (XII) & meningeal br of ascending pharyngeal art

INCISIVE CANAL
Site In ant maxilla extending from nose to incisive foramina
Contains Nasopalatine N, greater palatine vessels

INCISIVE FORAMEN
Site Midline, in ant hard palate. Openings of incisive canals into incisive fossa
Contains Nasopalatine N, greater palatine vessels

INCISIVE FOSSA (unpaired)
Site Median, in ant hard palate leading upwards to incisive foramina
Contains Nasopalatine Ns, greater palatine vessels

INFERIOR ORBITAL FISSURE
Site Between greater wing of sphenoid bone & maxilla
Contains Infra-orbital & zygomatic brs of maxillary N (Vb), infra-orbital vessels, inf ophthalmic Vs, orbital brs of pterygopalatine ganglion

INFRA-ORBITAL CANAL
Site Within orbital aspect of maxilla
Contains Infra-orbital N & vessels

INFRA-ORBITAL FORAMEN
Site Below infra-orbital margin in maxilla. Ant opening of infra-orbital canal
Contains Infra-orbital N & vessels

INTERNAL ACOUSTIC MEATUS
Site In post surface of petrous temporal bone in post cranial fossa

Contains Facial N (VII), nervus intermedius, vestibulocochlear N (VIII), labyrinthine art

INTERVERTEBRAL FORAMEN
Site Between vertebrae, bordered by—sup & inf: pedicles of vertebrae, ant: vertebral bodies & intervertebral disc, post: lig flavum covering sup & inf articular processes
Contains Spinal art & V, dorsal root ganglion, spinal N. Nerves C1–7 emerge via foramen above same numbered vertebra; nerve C8 exits below C7 vertebra & below this all nerves emerge via foramen below the same numbered vertebra

JUGULAR FORAMEN
Site Between jugular fossa of petrous temporal bone & occipital bone in post cranial fossa
Contains Glossopharyngeal N (IX), vagus (X), accessory N (XI), inf petrosal & sigmoid sinuses enters it, int jugular V emerges below

LESSER PALATINE FORAMINA
Site Two or three foramina in med & inf aspects of pyramidal process of palatine bone
Contains Lesser palatine Ns & vessels

MANDIBULAR CANAL (INFERIOR ALVEOLAR CANAL)
Site In body & ramus of mandible between mandibular & mental foramina
Contains Inf alveolar N & vessels

MANDIBULAR FORAMEN (INFERIOR ALVEOLAR FORAMEN)
Site Med aspect of ramus of mandible, overlapped anteromedially by lingula
Contains Inf alveolar N & vessels

MASTOID FORAMEN

Site In petrous temporal bone in post cranial fossa, post to sigmoid groove. Exits behind mastoid process

Contains Emissary V connecting sigmoid sinus & occipital Vs, meningeal br of occipital art

MENTAL FORAMEN

Site Outer aspect of ant ramus of mandible by second premolar tooth, leading from mandibular (inf alveolar) canal

Contains Mental N & vessels

NASOLACRIMAL CANAL

Site Between lacrimal bone & maxilla at ant/inf/med corner of orbit

Contains Nasolacrimal duct

OPTIC CANAL

Site In body of sphenoid bone in middle cranial fossa between body & two roots of lesser wing

Contains Optic N (II), dural sheath, ophthalmic art

PALATOVAGINAL CANAL

Site Between upper surface of sphenoidal process of palatine bone & lower surface of vaginal process of root of med ptery-goid plate in base of skull

Contains Pharyngeal Ns from maxillary (Vb) and pterygopalatine ganglion & pharyngeal br of maxillary art

PETROSQUAMOUS FISSURE

Site Between squamous temporal bone & tegmen tympani (petrous temporal bone)

Contains No structures

PETROTYMPANIC FISSURE

Site Between tympanic part (plate) of temporal bone & tegmen tympani (also part of temporal bone) in base of skull

Contains Chorda tympani, ant lig of malleus, ant tympanic br of maxillary art

PTERYGOID CANAL

Site In pterygoid process of sphenoid bone connecting ant wall of foramen lacerum to pterygopalatine fossa

Contains N & art of pterygoid canal

PTERYGOMAXILLARY FISSURE

Site Between lat pterygoid plate & post surface of maxilla connecting infra-temporal & pterygopalatine fossae, continuous above with post end of inf orbital fissure

Contains Terminal brs of maxillary art, passing in, post sup alveolar Ns passing out

SPHENOIDAL FORAMEN

Site In greater wing of sphenoid in middle cranial fossa med to foramen ovale (40% of skulls) (venous foramen of Vesalius)

Contains Emissary V connecting cavernous sinus & pterygoid plexus

SPHENOPALATINE FORAMEN

Site Between body of sphenoid bone & sphenopalatine notch of palatine bone (sup border of perpendicular plate & orbital & sphenoidal processes). In med wall of pterygopalatine fossa

Contains Sphenopalatine art, nasopalatine & sup nasal Ns from pterygopalatine fossa

SQUAMOTYMPANIC FISSURE

Site Between tympanic part (plate) of temporal bone & mandibular fossa (squamous temporal bone) in base of skull. It is divided by tegmen tympani (petrous temporal bone) into petro-tympanic and petrosquamous fissures

Contains Deep auricular br of maxillary artery

STYLOMASTOID FORAMEN
Site Between styloid & mastoid processes of temporal bone in base of skull
Contains Facial N (VII) & stylomastoid br of post auricular art

SUPERIOR ORBITAL FISSURE
Site Between body & lesser & greater wings of sphenoid bone in middle cranial fossa
Contains Ophthalmic N (Va) (lacrimal, frontal, nasociliary brs), ophthalmic Vs, oculomotor N (sup & inf divs) (III), trochlear N (IV), abducent N (VI), sympathetic fibres, brs of middle meningeal & lacrimal arts

SUPRA-ORBITAL FORAMEN
Site In supra-orbital margin of frontal bone, 2 cm from midline
Contains Supra-orbital N & vessels

VERTEBRAL FORAMEN (unpaired)
Site Bordered by—ant: body of vertebra, post: laminae, lat: pedicles & articular processes. Collectively making the spinal canal
Contains Spinal cord/cauda equina, dura, archnoid & pia mater, cerebrospinal fluid, internal vertebral venous plexus & spinal arts

VOMEROVAGINAL CANAL
Site Between lower aspect of ala of vomer & upper aspect of vaginal process of root of med pterygoid plate in base of skull (not always present)
Contains Pharyngeal br of sphenopalatine art

ZYGOMATICOFACIAL FORAMEN
Site In lat surface of zygomatic bone
Contains Zygomaticofacial N & vessels

ZYGOMATICO-ORBITAL FORAMEN
Site In orbital surface of zygomatic bone
Contains Zygomatic br of maxillary N (Vb)

ZYGOMATICOTEMPORAL FORAMEN
Site In posteromedial surface of zygomatic bone
Contains Zygomaticotemporal N & vessels

11

12: SPACES OTHER THAN SKULL AND SPINE

Notes: (1) Including fossae, spaces, rings, canals, triangles, sacs and foramina. (2) All paired unless otherwise indicated.

12

ADDUCTOR (HUNTER'S/SUBSARTORIAL) CANAL

Site A groove in thigh extending from apex of femoral triangle to hiatus in adductor magnus. Bordered by—lat: vastus medialis, med: adductor longus & magnus, roof: fascia in which lies the subsartorial plexus & on which lies sartorius

Contains Femoral art & vein; saphenous N; N to vastus medialis

ANTERIOR TRIANGLE OF NECK

Site Borders—inf border of mandible, midline & ant border of sternocleidomastoid. Subdivided into carotid, digastric, submental & muscular triangles

Contains Muscles: digastric, stylohyoid, mylohyoid, geniohyoid, sternohyoid, omohyoid, thyrohyoid, sternothyroid, platysma. Hyoid bone, larynx, thyroid & parathyroid glands, trachea, oesophagus, submandibular gland, lymph nodes. Arteries: common, int & ext carotids; brs of ext carotid: sup thyroid, ascending pharyngeal, lingual, facial (submental). Mylohyoid art (maxillary via inf alveolar). Veins: int & ant jugular. Nerves: hypoglossal, ansa cervicalis, vagus & its int, ext & recurrent laryngeal & pharyngeal brs, mylohyoid N from Vc via inf alveolar N

CUBITAL FOSSA

Site Triangular space in ant aspect of arm. Borders—sup: intercondylar line, med: lat border of pronator teres, lat: med border of brachioradialis, floor: brachialis, supinator, roof: fascia (see below for what lies in it)

Contains From med to lat: median N, brachial art & its accompanying Vs, biceps tendon, radial & post interosseous Ns seen under edge of brachioradialis. Roof: bicipital aponeurosis, median basilic & cephalic Vs, med & lat cutaneous Ns of forearm

DEEP INGUINAL RING

Site A defect in transversalis fascia in lower abdominal wall above mid point of inguinal lig. Borders—sup & lat: curved fibres of transversus abdominis. Inf: inguinal lig. Med: transversalis fascia & inf epigastric vessels. Int spermatic fascia attached to its edges

Contains Vas deferens; testicular, vasal, cremasteric arts & Vs; obliterated processus vaginalis; genital br of genitofemoral N; autonomic Ns; lymphatics

EPIPLOIC FORAMEN OF WINSLOW (ADITUS TO LESSER SAC) (unpaired)

Site In upper abdomen. Borders—ant: portal V, bile duct & hepatic art in free edge of lesser omentum, post: inf vena cava, inf: first part of duodenum, sup: caudate lobe of liver

Contains Nil

FEMORAL RING & CANAL

Site In lower abdomen. Femoral ring is upper end of femoral canal. Borders—ant: inguinal lig, med: lacunar lig, post: pectineal lig & pectineus, lat: femoral V

Contains Cloquet's node; lymphatics

FEMORAL TRIANGLE

Site In ant thigh. Borders—med: med border of adductor longus, lat: med border of sartorius, sup: inguinal lig, floor: adductor longus, pectineus, iliacus & psoas, roof: fascia lata

Contains Femoral N, art, V & their brs; deep inguinal lymph nodes

GREATER SCIATIC FORAMEN

Site In pelvis between greater sciatic notch of ischium/ilium & both sacrotuberous & sacrospinous ligs

Contains From above downwards: sup gluteal N & vessels, piriformis, inf gluteal N & vessels, int pudendal art, pudendal N, sciatic N, post femoral cutaneous N,

12

perforating cutaneous N, N to obturator internus, N to quadratus femoris

INGUINAL CANAL

Site In lower abdomen between deep & superficial inguinal rings. Borders—ant: external oblique abdominis & a small portion of internal oblique abdominis, post: transversalis fascia, inf epigastric vessels & conjoint tendon, sup: curved fibres of internal oblique & transversus abdominis, inf: inguinal lig

Contains Vas deferens/round lig of uterus; testicular, cremasteric & vasal arts & Vs; obliterated processus vaginalis; ilio-inguinal, genital br of genitofemoral & autonomic Ns; lymphatics; int spermatic & cremasteric fasciae

INGUINAL (HASSELBACH'S) TRIANGLE

Site Post aspect of ant abdominal wall in inguinal region. Borders—lat: inf epigastric art, med: lat edge of rectus abdominis, inf: inguinal lig, floor: transversalis fascia, conjoint tendon & post wall of inguinal canal

Contains Nil. Site of direct inguinal herniation

ISCHIO-ANAL (ISCHIORECTAL) FOSSA

Site Wedge-shaped area lat to anal canal. Borders—med: anal canal & levator ani, lat: obturator internus & ischial tuberosity, inf (floor/base): post aspect of perineal body, urogenital diaphragm, sacrotuberous lig & gluteus maximus

Contains Fat; pudendal canal containing pudendal N & int pudendal vessels; inf rectal N & vessels as brs of above

LATERAL TRIANGULAR SPACE

Site In post wall of axilla. Borders— sup/med: teres major, inf/med: long head of triceps, lat: med shaft of humerus

Contains Radial N; profunda brachii vessels

LESSER SAC (OMENTAL BURSA)

(unpaired)

Site Diverticulum from general peritoneal cavity in upper abdomen opening via epiploic foramen of Winslow

Contains Its peritoneal lining lies against— ant (from above down): post surface of liver; lesser omentum; body & fundus of stomach; greater omentum. Inf: transverse colon. Post: inf vena cava; first 2.5 cm of duodenum; aorta; coeliac trunk & brs; body of pancreas; left suprarenal gland; upper pole left kidney; sup: caudate lobe of liver; med (right): opening of sac with inf vena cava in post edge; portal V, hepatic art & bile duct in ant free edge; lat (left): gastrosplenic & lienorenal ligs with spleen between them

LESSER SCIATIC FORAMEN

Site In pelvis between lesser sciatic notch of ischium & both sacrotuberous & sacrospinous ligs

Contains Passing out: tendon of obturator internus & int. pudendal V. Passing in: N to obturator internus, int pudendal art, pudendal N

MEDIAL TRIANGULAR SPACE

Site In post wall of axilla. Borders— sup/med: subscapularis (teres minor viewed from behind), inf/lat: teres major, lat: long head of triceps

Contains Circumflex scapular art

OBTURATOR CANAL

Site In ant aspect of obturator foramen in lat wall of true pelvis. Borders—ant: post public ramus, sup/inf/med: obturator int & its fascia

Contains Obturator N & vessels

POPLITEAL FOSSA

Site Diamond shaped, behind knee. Borders—sup/lat: biceps femoris, sup/med: semitendinosus & semimembranosus, inf/med & inf/lat:

12

heads of gastrocnemius, floor: post distal femur, post capsule of knee & popliteus, roof: fascia

Contains Plantaris; popliteal art & V & brs; tibial, common peroneal, sural & sural communicating Ns; lymph nodes & fat. Short saphenous V & post femoral cutaneous N in fascia of roof

POSTERIOR TRIANGLE OF NECK

Site Between post border of sternocleidomastoid, ant border of trapezius & middle third of clavicle. Floor: prevertebral fascia over semispinalis capitis, splenius capitis, levator scapulae, scalenus medius & ant. Roof: investing layer of deep fascia

Contains Occipital, transverse cervical, suprascapular & third part of subclavian arts; transverse cervical, suprascapular & ext jugular Vs; muscular & cutaneous brs of cervical plexus (lesser occipital, great auricular, transverse cervical, supraclavicular); three trunks of brachial plexus; spinal root of accessory N; inf belly of omohyoid; superficial cervical lymph nodes

PUDENDAL (ALCOCK'S) CANAL

Site Lies within a fascial sheath in lat wall of ischio-anal fossa between lesser sciatic notch & deep perineal pouch. Borders— lat: obturator internus & ischial tuberosity, med: fat

Contains Pudendal N; int pudendal vessels

QUADRANGULAR SPACE

Site In post wall of axilla. Borders—sup: subscapularis (teres minor viewed from behind), inf: teres major, med: long head of triceps, lat: med shaft of humerus

Contains Axillary N; post circumflex humeral art & V

SNUFF BOX

Site A triangular depression on dorsolateral side of hand formed by tendons of extensor pollicis longus (ulnar side) & extensor pollicis brevis & abductor pollicis longus (radial side)

Contains Scaphoid, trapezium, radial art; terminal brs of radial N pass over it

SUPERFICIAL INGUINAL RING

Site In lower abdominal wall at med end of inguinal canal as a V-shaped opening of ext oblique aponeurosis. Ext spermatic fascia is attached to its edges

Contains In female: ilio-inguinal N & round lig of uterus. In males: ilio-inguinal N & spermatic cord (vas deferens; testicular, cremasteric & vasal arts & Vs; obliterated processus vaginalis; genital br of genitofemoral & autonomic Ns; lymphatics; int spermatic & cremasteric fasciae)

UROGENITAL TRIANGLE

Site In perineum. Borders—lat: ischiopubic rami, ant: post aspect of symphysis pubis, post: transverse line at level of perineal body & ischial tuberosities

Contains Deep perineal pouch (space) within sup & inf fascial layers of the urogenital diaphragm perforated by urethra with surrounding ext sphincter; deep transverse perinei; brs of int pudendal vessels & pudendal N. In male diaphragm contains bulbo-urethral glands & supports penis, scrotum & superficial transverse perinei from its inf surface. In female it is perforated by vagina

2

13: POSITION OF STRUCTURES ACCORDING TO VERTEBRAL LEVELS

Notes: (1) A /(oblique stroke) between two levels indicates that the structure lies at a level between these two vertebrae. (2) A — (dash) between two levels indicates that the structure occupies the equivalent level to these vertebrae inclusively.

C1 Spinal root of accessory nerve crosses transverse process of atlas
Open mouth and dens

C2 Superior cervical ganglion

C3 Body of hyoid bone

C4 Upper border of thyroid cartilage
Bifurcation of common carotid arteries

C6 Cricoid cartilage
Larynx becomes trachea
Pharynx becomes oesophagus
Middle cervical ganglion
Vertebral artery enters foramen transversarium of C6 vertebra
Carotid tubercle of Chassaignac
Inferior thyroid artery crosses to thyroid gland

C7 First clearly palpable spinous process (vertebra prominens)
Stellate/inferior cervical ganglion

T2 Superior border of scapula

T2/3 Suprasternal notch

T3 Medial end of spine of scapula
End of oblique fissure of lung posteriorly at spine of T3

T3/4 Top of arch of aorta

T3–4 Manubrium sterni

T4 End of arch of aorta
Azygos vein enters superior vena cava

T4/5 Manubriosternal angle of Louis
Bifurcation of trachea
Start of arch of aorta

T5 Thoracic duct crosses midline

T5–8 Sternum

T6 Upper border of liver

T7 Inferior angle of scapula
Accessory hemiazygos vein crosses midline to azygos vein

T8 Caval opening in diaphragm
• Inferior vena cava
• Right phrenic nerve
Left phrenic nerve pierces diaphragm lat to central tendon
Hemiazygos vein crosses to right to join azygos vein

T8/9 Sternoxiphisternal joint

T9 Superior epigastic vessels traverse diaphragm
Xiphoid

T10 Oesophageal opening in diaphragm
• Oesophagus
• Brs of left gastric vessels
• Anterior and posterior vagi

T12 Aortic 'opening' in diaphragm posterior to median arcuate lig
• Aorta
• Azygos & hemiazygos veins
• Thoracic duct
Origin of coeliac axis (lower bo... of T12)

Splanchnic nerves pierce crura of diaphragm

Sympathetic trunk passes posterior to medial arcuate ligament

Subcostal neurovascular bundle passes posterior to lateral arcuate lig

L1   Transpyloric plane of Addison (half way between suprasternal notch and symphysis pubis)
- Fundus of gallbladder
- Hila of kidneys
- Second part of duodenum
- Neck of pancreas
- Origin of superior mesenteric artery
- Origin of portal vein
- Pylorus
- Attachment of transverse mesocolon
- Hilum of spleen (spleen on ribs 9, 10, 11)
- Tip of 9th costal cartilage

L1/2   Origin of renal arteries
Spinal cord ends in adults

L2   Subcostal plane
- Formation of azygos and hemiazygos veins
- Duodenojejunal flexure, ligament of Treitz (upper border of L2)

L3   Origin of inferior mesenteric artery

L3/4   Umbilicus

L4   Supracristal plane (iliac crests)
- Bifurcation of aorta

L5   Formation of inferior vena cava

S2   Sacral dimple
Mid point of sacro-iliac joint
Post superior iliac spine
Dural sac ends

S3   Start of rectum

S4   Sacral hiatus
End of vertebral canal

Co1   Filum terminale inserts

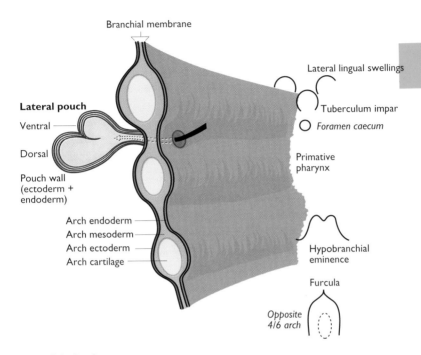

Branchial membrane

Lateral lingual swellings

Tuberculum impar

Foramen caecum

Lateral pouch

Ventral

Dorsal

Pouch wall
(ectoderm +
endoderm)

Arch endoderm
Arch mesoderm
Arch ectoderm
Arch cartilage

Primative
pharynx

Hypobranchial
eminence

Furcula

Opposite
4/6 arch

Pharyngeal derivatives

Pharyngeal derivatives

Arch	Arch derivatives		Endoderm	Lateral pouch derivatives		Artery	Nerve
	Cartilages, bones, ligaments (Mesoderm)	Muscles		Endoderm	Ectoderm		
1 'Mandibular' arch cartilage = Meckel's	Incus Malleus Anterior lig of malleus Sphenomandibular lig (Lingula) (Mandible*)	Masseter Temporalis Pterygoids Mylohyoid Anterior belly of digastric Tensor veli palatini Tensor tympani	Mucous membrane & glands of anterior 2/3 of tongue	Auditory tube Inner layer of tympanic membrane (Part of middle ear) (Mastoid antrum)	External acoustic meatus Outer layer of tympanic membrane (Tragus of ear) (Skin of lower face)	Part of maxillary artery	Mandibular division of trigeminal (Vc)
2 'Hyoid' arch cartilage = Reichert's	Upper body & lesser cornu of hyoid Stylohyoid ligament Styloid process Stapes	Stapedius Stylohyoid Posterior belly of digastric Muscles of facial expression including buccinator & platysma	—	Supratonsillar fossa Tonsillar crypts Surface epithelium of tonsil** (Part of middle ear)	Overgrowth of ectoderm over arches 3, 4 & 6	Stapedial artery	Facial (VII)

14

Arch		Skeletal	Muscles	Mucous membrane	Pouch derivatives		Artery	Nerve
3	'Thyrohyoid' arch	Inferior body & greater cornu of hyoid	Stylopharyngeus	Mucous membrane & glands of posterior 1/3 of tongue	Ventral: epithelial cells of thymus**; Dorsal: inferior parathyroid	—	Internal carotid artery (including carotid sinus)	Glossopharyngeal (IX)
4		Thyroid cartilage	Palatoglossus, Palatopharyngeus, Salpingopharyngeus, Cricothyroid, Levator veli palatini, Striated of oesophagus, Pharyngeal constrictors	Valleculae & anterior epiglottis	Ventral: ultimobranchial bodies†; Dorsal: superior parathyroid	—	Right: part of right subclavian artery; Left: aortic arch	Vagus (X) Pharyngeal & superior laryngeal branches
6		Cricoid cartilage, Vocal ligs, Arytenoid, corniculate & cuneiform cartilages	Cricopharyngeus, All intrinsic muscles of larynx	—	Lung buds	—	Ventral: pulmonary artery; Dorsal: ductus arteriosus	Vagus (X) Recurrent laryngeal branch

* The mandible forms in membrane around the ventral aspect of the first arch cartilage.

** The lymphoid tissue of the tonsil and thymus arises from the surrounding mesenchyme and is not arch derivative.

† Ultimobranchial bodies develop from ventral parts of fourth (and possibly fifth) pouch and fuse with the developing thyroid to give parafollicular (C) cells which produce calcitonin.

Notes: (1) The thyroid gland arises from between the first and second arch as a diverticulum (thyroglossal duct) which grows downwards leaving the foramen caecum at its origin. (2) The epiglottis comes from the inferior part of the hypobranchial eminence and is thus not a true arch derivative. (3) Bracketed information is of additional interest.

14